Building a Results-Based Student Support Program

SHARON JOHNSON
California State University, Los Angeles

CLARENCE JOHNSON
Walden University

LOUIS DOWNS
California State University, Sacramento

Lahaska Press
Houghton Mifflin Company
Boston   New York

Publisher, Lahaska Press: Barry Fetterolf
Senior Editor, Lahaska Press: Mary Falcon
Editorial Assistant: Lindsey Gentel
Senior Project Editor: Kathryn Dinovo
Senior Manufacturing Buyer: Renee Ostrowski
Marketing Manager: Barbara LeBuhn-Maly

Cover image: © Royalty-Free/Corbis

Lahaska Press was established as an imprint of Houghton Mifflin Company in 1999. It is dedicated to publishing textbooks and instructional media for counseling and the helping professions. The editorial offices of the imprint are located in the small town of Lahaska, Pennsylvania. "Lahaska" is a Native American Lenape word meaning "source of much writing."

Printed in the U.S.A.

Library of Congress Control Number: 2005927118

ISBN: 0-618-54336-8

123456789-VHO-09 08 07 06 05

Contents

Appendixes   177

Preface

The purpose of this manual is to assist readers in developing a set of professional competencies that lead to the establishment of a results-based student support program. It uses a step-by-step workbook approach to present each element within the results-based student support program. The manual is designed for use by students in graduate school counseling courses as well as by practicing school counselors who are making the shift from traditional counseling services to student support programs. To clarify terminology, we will use the word *students* to refer to K–12 students, and *you* or *class members* to refer to readers/users of this text. Activities are designed for simulated or actual teams/groups, working together from diverse perspectives. We believe that the only way to learn collaboration skills is within a group context, and because a student support team includes members from a variety of disciplines, collaboration, listening, and consensus become important skills in the process. However, the group design of the activities does not preclude for the use of this text by individuals in a college class.

The approach we advocate in this book is a shift away from the notion of guidance (student support) programs as services offered by counselors and other student support personnel. The new focus ensures that students acquire pre-determined competencies. Any change takes time, and this change of focus has taken a long time to be accepted by many educators. Historically, the shift from services-oriented school counseling programs to student-centered results-based efforts gained momentum with the realization that as the focus of education changes, student support programs must also change. The prevailing myth in school counseling was, and still is in many places, that counselors graduate from colleges and universities with masters' degrees and the belief they will be hired to work individually and in small groups with students to help solve students' problems and successfully address their developmental concerns. But a newly hired school counselor soon discovers the truth: that school counselors and other student support staff are hired as educators to teach students skills needed for academic, career, social, and personal success. The myth of defining guidance in terms of "what counselors do" has been gradually replaced by the question "How are students different because of the student support program?" This shift to program and individual accountability for results in school guidance is not new (Gysbers, 2003). What is new is a systemic approach that aligns the guidance curriculum with other school curricula. Also new is the fact that the results-based approach is no longer looked upon as an auxiliary effort; it functions an equal partner with other subject areas and other student support disciplines (school psychology, school social work, nurses, and others) to ensure that students acquire and demonstrate identified program goals and specific competencies related to the mission of schools, namely, academic achievement.

The results-based student support program was developed over a period of time beginning in 1972. Based on the systemic educational paradigm of Roger Kaufman (1968), it consists of ends (results) and means (resources and activities). Management of activities is performed by the person accountable for the results. That is, counselors and other student support personnel accountable for specific results are in charge of those activities, including the resources. This means that student support professionals must have competencies in leadership, including planning, managing, collecting, and using data to improve the processes, and in monitoring individual student's academic and social development progress.

Results-based student support programs require creating new ways to ensure that each student acquires the desired competencies. Traditionally, counselors found themselves spending 90% of their time with 10% of the students. Now they will shift to spending 90% of their time with 90% of the students. To accomplish this goal, student support professionals need to give up some of their current work activities and look for new methods that will impact all the students. They will have to take leadership in program development, maintenance, and evaluation. The change might call for student support personnel to develop or renew leadership skills, including collaborating and student advocacy, conducting in-service activities, involving parent and community in the guidance process, and leading group processes such as conducting meetings, counseling, and conducting guidance groups.

The exercises in this workbook are designed to provide readers with ample opportunity to acquire knowledge-based, skill-based, and attitudinal competencies. Upon completion of the exercises in this book, readers should be able to demonstrate the following knowledge-based competencies:

1. Know the differences between services and results-based programs

2. Know the linkages among systems, results, resources, and management

3. Possess skills in developing the program results—mission, philosophy, goals, and related competencies

4. Possess skills in collaborating with others to reach mutual goals

5. Appreciate others' skills, attitudes, and contributions

6. Know personal competencies that match the requirements for developing and implementing a results-based student support program

They should also be able to demonstrate the following skill-based competencies:

1. Know the reciprocal administrator-personnel management system

2. Use consensus in making decisions

3. Know the benefits of using results agreements

4. Prepare a results agreement at a specific grade level

5. Recognize needs data related to students' academic and social development

6. Complete results plans

7. Understand advocacy processes that might be used in monitoring students' academic, career, personal, and social development

8. Use data to enhance an ongoing program as well effecting change within the system

9. Know the importance of, and possess skills in, developing a one-year program calendar

10. Know the importance of and the skill required to develop and implement a results-based guidance or student support program

And finally, they should acquire the following attitudinal competencies:

1. Know the research on how parent involvement in their children's education affects the children's academic and social development

2. Appreciate the freedom allowed in using their results agreements to decide their own contributions to students

3. Acquire skills in brainstorming, and preparing for and conducting meetings

4. Use benchmarks and school profile information to monitor students' development

5. Appreciate consultation opportunities

6. Appreciate others' differences and contributions to the development (and implementation) of a comprehensive results-based program that interfaces with each and every student in the school

Acknowledgments

Developing the conceptual systemic results-based model for student support personnel took commitment by others who believed in the model and moved ahead, having faith in the concept but with no proven formula. These pioneers discovered that they had greater control over implementation of their programs, but their most important discovery was the realization that the results-based model itself had to be adapted to their own school community culture. They also learned that the right way to get the program started was not to be found in any formula or predictable sequence. There were also leaders in the field who took steps in parallel efforts, sharing the same vision but forging their own trails. Only in the last few years have all these efforts come together in a comprehensive agreement that students are the primary clients and student results need to be the primary focus of student support efforts.

We extend our appreciation to the hundreds of school-based counselors, directors of guidance, and other professionals who have successfully implemented the results-based guidance program. They are the professionals who need recognition for their day-by-day efforts to ensure that each student leaves school with the necessary competencies to make a successful transition to higher education, employment, or a combination of work and education. This text reflects the efforts of many of our colleagues who have provided feedback, arguing for and against the ideas in an effort to come to consensus, and who are moving ahead in the face of a myriad of problems confronting schools and students.

We specifically thank the following colleagues for their efforts and honesty in reviewing the first draft of this textbook: Fred Bemak, George Mason University; Joyce DeVoss, Northern Arizona University; Tamara Davis, Marymount University; Russell Sabella, Florida Gulf Coast University; Christopher Sink, Seattle Pacific University; Brent Snow, State University of West Georgia; Diane Talbot, California State University-Fresno; and Sandra Zimmerman, Sonoma State University.

PART ONE

Introduction and Background

CHAPTER ONE

Introduction to Results-Based Student Support

Upon completion of this chapter and its activities, you should be able to demonstrate the following competencies:

- **Summarize the history of school counseling and guidance**
- **Understand the major differences between the new results-based student support program model and the traditional process-based services model of guidance**

▪ *Introduction*

"What do counselors do?" This perennial question continues to drive the actions and communication of counselors in schools across the nation. Although education has undergone numerous changes—especially since the 1980s, when the reform in education movement became most pronounced—most student support programs have kept the same services within a traditional model. In fact, few of the recent educational reform studies address student support programs, and school-based in-service programs frequently omit counselors.

■ *Background*

One of the important antecedents to current trends in counseling and guidance was the passage of the National Defense Education Act (NDEA) in 1958. This legislation reaffirmed and extended the role of school counselors as a part of massive efforts in school reform. The focus of this effort was to identify and encourage able high school students to study sciences and mathematics and to continue these studies in college. The provisions of this act had profound and positive effects on the number of school counselors, the availability of counselor education programs, the development of a professional literature in school counseling, the organization of K–12 programs of school guidance, and the commitment of state departments of education to increase the certification requirements for school counselors.

A second important legislative thrust for school counseling was the Manpower Development and Training Act of 1962 and the Vocational Education Act of 1963. These and other pieces of legislation focused school reform on workforce preparation and vocational guidance and counseling.

As early as 1972, the current movement from counseling services to comprehensive results-based programs was introduced as a way to help all students achieve. The drive to focus all educational resources toward academic achievement as measured by standardized test scores swept the national political scene in the late 1990s and early 2000s. "No Child Left Behind" was the impetus for using federal and state funds as rewards and withdrawal of funds as punishment for schools and districts based on the level of student achievement and/or improvement based primarily on test scores.

For the most part, student support programs have received little attention in the quest for higher academic standards, state mandated testing, and rigorous graduation requirements. Regular training and retraining for administrators and teachers is now expected, but there has been little or no in-service provision for student support professionals. The educational community has neglected to address the importance of providing the support that students need to achieve the new standards. Student support programs essentially have stayed the same, with elements added to adjust to new teaching and administration models.

The time for change in traditional guidance and counseling programs is imminent. Students are being pressured to attain new heights of academic achievement in order to graduate, to attend a college, to prepare for a new job market, to reach escalating standards in every area. However, few resources are available to ensure they gain the skills in learning and working that are necessary for their success, and even fewer resources to help deal with the added stress in their lives and the environment. Because of financial constraints caused by years of political rhetoric and budget cuts, schools have large classroom teacher-pupil ratios as well as large counselor-student ratios. The concept of downsizing (i.e., doing more with less) has led to even greater responsibilities for already overloaded student support personnel.

The Add-on Student Support Model

The "add-on" model is the result of reactive guidance programs and lack of leadership in pupil personnel programs. Guidance programs were initially established to help students match their skills with available job options. This period was followed by the "add-on" of mental health counseling. Next came a move to emphasize college and university placement along with assistance in helping students find financial aid. The mission of NDEA-V was to educate counselors to advise more students to take science and math. The result of these trends was the development of programs to prepare counselors to do primarily individual and group counseling. In the 1960s, counselors were admonished to lower student dropout rates; in the 1970s, they were career development and educational specialists; and in the 1980s, they were called upon to be drug and child abuse prevention specialists. During the 1970s and 1980s, the add-ons (Aubrey, 1985) included helping children cope with broken families and alienation from adult society, economic downsizing, and AIDS. Yet another major add-on became helping students and their parents to cope with a rapidly changing society. Responsibilities continue to be added and few are deleted, even though parents and students continue to press counselors for more answers on how to get into a university or college, how to access financial aid, how to keep students off drugs and alcohol, how to motivate students to stay in school and increase their learning, and how to help parents set up learning rituals in the home.

The newest and perhaps most challenging add-ons have to do with student health and safety within the schools. School violence and bullying have risen to crisis proportions along with the requisite need to teach students new skills in protecting themselves from physical harm. Other increasingly prominent problems include the increase in student obesity, high blood pressure, diabetes, stress, and self-mutilation as well as other health-related problems that interfere with learning.

Recent Counseling and Guidance Trends

In the early 1980s, a model was developed in Huntington Beach, California, that replaced counselors with guidance technicians trained to do scheduling and record keeping. Career development became a classroom teacher's responsibility, and a single school psychologist was used to address the needs of students with serious emotional and learning problems. College and career fairs, when offered, were coordinated by central office staff and held during evening hours. Other guidance-related needs of students were not formally addressed. This trend has been replicated in schools throughout the United States as more districts look to this model when their budgets are slashed and reduction of budgets becomes the highest priority. In many cases, volunteers or paraprofessionals are given the title "counselor," and parents, teachers, and students are unaware of their lack of training and credentials. The same board members who approve these measures, paradoxically, would be aghast if volunteers were put into the classroom and called "teachers." Researchers (Kasler, 1989) found some similarities between the functions of guidance technicians and credentialed counselors, but reported that counselors tended to be more competent in delivering counseling services.

Another model, called *guaranteed guidance services* (White, 1981) also emerged in the early 1980s. This approach guaranteed that counselors would provide specific services such as college and career planning, individual and group counseling, and test administration. Although this model was very popular in California in the 1980s and 1990s, it has been discontinued in most venues. One major problem with providing services in this way is that the accountability and evaluation rest in user satisfaction surveys, indications of how much time is spent on specific tasks, a count of number of processes completed, and number of students served. These data reflect how counselors spend their time but show little indication of the impact of the services on the students.

Teacher-advisor and mentoring programs (Myrick & Myrick, 1990) have reemerged and are gaining support as an alternative delivery system. This approach holds the teacher-advisors or mentors accountable for certain guidance results, while counselors handle added-on duties. In fact, some school systems have implemented the teacher-advisor program almost to the exclusion of counselors (Bradley, 1986; Myrick & Myrick, 1992), while others make counselors responsible for developing the program but not for direct counseling duties (Henderson, 1989). New mentoring programs have emphasized the need for a more collaborative approach in which teachers, community agencies, parents, and student support staff work together to define, deliver, and assess student achievement. One example of this type of program (Gallassi & Gulledge, 1997), a version of the Teacher Advisor Program (TAP), blended the roles of teacher and counselor. An inherent risk for counselors in this model is that the assumption that the teacher is the guidance advisor is so strong that Gallassi and Gulledge, who described the program for *Professional School Counseling*, felt the need to defend the very existence of counselors themselves. The advisor/mentor assumes the responsibility for regular monitoring of student attainment of educational competencies.

An increasingly popular development is the comprehensive guidance model (Gysbers & Henderson, 1988), which began as a career development model for the Missouri schools. This approach includes a variety of elements including guidance curriculum and individual and group counseling. Accountability includes how much time counselors spend on guidance-related activities as well as on providing system support. New additions to this model include delineation of leadership skills needed by counselors to ensure program implementation and accountability. An interesting variant on the Missouri comprehensive guidance model blends this model and the teacher-advisor model of service delivery (Walz, 1992), in which the actual duties are carefully defined between counselor and teacher, but counselors are relegated to add-on duties.

A new model of the 1990s defined guidance as a community responsibility in which parents, businesses, government agencies, organizations, and school personnel all contribute to guiding and counseling youth (Herr, 1989). Although funding was available to implement this model, it faded quickly from view and was discontinued in most districts by the late 1990s. Still, models continue to be developed in an effort to increase the community's involvement and investment in education. Stone and Dyal (1997) reported on one school program that heavily involved parents with teachers to deliver the bulk of guidance curricula, including personal-social interventions in the classroom. An alternative approach (Rowley, Sink, & MacDonald, 2002) also involved parents heavily in the personal-social domain of counseling but defined a distinct and extensive role for school counselors as well. Another model, developed statewide in Maine and New Hampshire, used counselors as leaders in collaboration with community members to deliver career guidance services (Hayslip, 2000). Contrary to models of community-school collaboration that reduce counselor involvement, Bemak (2000) posited not only a significant role for counselors in a collaborative guidance program but also a more expansive view of community involvement. Based on the premise that school counselors should also be social change agents and that students will only do well if they and their environments are healthy physically and psychologically, the model reflects involvement of mental health, public health, and other community entities seldom mentioned in other community-school collaboration literature. This extension of the definition of community involvement is in keeping with federal legislation (HR 5, 1997) that requires mental health agencies to service schools. It also sets the stage for the School and Family Integration Model (Bemak & Cornely, 2002), which uses the expanded resources to link schools with marginalized families.

Another perspective is found in a counselor retraining model, *mentoring*, which calls for experienced counselors to work closely with new colleagues to provide in-service training and to teach new skills (Anderson, 1989). Ancillary to this model is a trend that focuses on career ladders/lattices (Johnson, 1987; Steinberg, 1988) that encompass differential staffing to make more effective use of individual counselors' skills. This scaffolding has worked best with programs that concentrate the bulk of their guidance emphasis on the career domain (Beale, 2001; Jarvis & Keeley, 2003; Ireh, 2000).

An emerging paradigm that identifies the student as the primary client and designs all reform efforts in terms of the results for students is the comprehensive *results-based student support program* model (Johnson & Johnson, 1998). This program is designed as a systemic approach that integrates the program into the educational experience of each student. It ensures equity to guarantee that *all* students acquire the competencies to become successful in school and to make a successful transition from school to higher education, employment, or a combination of higher education and work. It addresses the three domains (education, occupation, and personal-social) that were identified in the National Study of Guidance Taxonomy of Objectives developed by Frank Wellman in 1962. These same domains are used as the foundation for the ASCA National Standards (1997). Lapan's (2001) argument in support of comprehensive results-based guidance programs laid a further philosophical base for justifying a model to develop student cognitive competence and aligning school counseling with the developmental theories of Super and Seligman.

With the publication of national standards and a national model for school counseling programs (2003), the American School Counselor Association (ASCA) has generated another important trend. These publications, based on the work of theorists in the counseling field, articulate the need for counselors to provide programs designed for student success in the academic, career, and personal-social domains. The ASCA national model, building on models developed by Norm Gysbers, C. D. and S. K. Johnson, and Robert Myrick, has been effective in increasing the visibility and the credibility of school counselors. However, it does not define accountability measures for student results, as does the results-based student support.

New on the scene is the Transforming Counselor Education project, funded by the Education Trust and MetLife Foundation (Martin & House, 1998). This effort to address advocacy for students seeks to place practicing school counselors at the heart of the new mission of schools, which is to educate all students to reach high academic standards. This project has more fully utilized the idea of "data-driven" programs than previous models. Counselors are trained in collecting and utilizing data to identify target areas and then plan and implement specific approaches to address the most pressing concerns within a school (House & Hayes, 2002). However, the strong emphasis on counselor intervention dedicated to academic development of students may in some cases limit guidance program responsibilities in the personal-social and career domains. Both the Transforming Counselor Education project and the results-based student support model have generated greater data-driven program development. Isaacs (2003) strongly stated the need for better preparation of counselors' research capabilities if data-driven program development is to become a reality.

Paradigm Shift

Education is being newly conceptualized. "Under the old conceptualization, education was thought of as process and system, effort and intention, investment and hope. To improve education meant to try harder, to engage in more activity, to magnify one's plans, to give people more services, and to become more efficient in delivering them" (Finn, 1990, p. 586). Similarly, the old model of traditional guidance emphasized the position and duties of the counselor or the therapeutic process of counseling at the expense of a coherent programmatic focus. Consequently, guidance has been widely regarded as an ancillary support service rather than as an integral part of education. Joel Barker (1987), reviewing Kuhn's (1970) work on paradigm shifts, indicated that one's perspective on a given subject serves as a screen or filter, making it impossible at times to see conflicting information clearly. It may be this phenomenon that has kept us from recognizing the need to reconceptualize the guidance field, reframing it in a new light.

The quality of an organization can be judged by the quality of the questions its members choose to answer. "The important element in decision making is defining the question" (Drucker, 1971). Guidance professionals have spent many years trying to define school counseling by answering the wrong question. The question, "What do counselors do?" leads us in an endless circle of describing a variety of processes and services available to students and staff. As these processes change, the answer to the prevailing question has to be readdressed to respond to our many publics. The new paradigm question to answer is, "How are students different as a result of the student support program?" Clearly, if students do not benefit from a guidance program by acquiring new knowledge or skills, then there is little, if any, need or reason to continue the program. The following are some contrasts between traditional add-on counseling programs and the new comprehensive, results-based programs.

Focus on Student Results The results-based approach is a comprehensive, developmental student support program based on students' need for competencies in learning, working, relating, and leading a balanced, healthful lifestyle. The difference between this approach and add-on services is a basic difference in philosophy between offering students an opportunity to experience and benefit from guidance at their own request (services model) or providing a planned, sequential program in which counselors take responsibility for assuring that each student gains specific guidance-related competencies. *Services* have traditionally been based on student demand and local school need. *Competencies* are based on professionally identified educational, career, personal, and social needs of students.

The importance of this distinction is evident when one looks at the credibility of school counseling within the total educational program. The traditional focus on defined activities and process provides little relationship to education reform, little proof of effectiveness, and little justification to expand the number of counselors when the focus of education is on reaching state and federal mandates while dealing with massive budgetary cutbacks.

Accountability Accountability is now focused on student results. Traditionally, accountability in guidance amounted to a role and function statement to define counselor duties, approximate the amount of time spent on each function, and count the number of students going through a process. In a results-based student support program, it is assumed that students learn differently and a variety of processes are required to ensure success for all students. In traditional programs, specific processes are established for all counselors and so only a percentage of students can be expected to attain the desired competencies. In the results-based program, data collection, analysis, and reflection on results are done on a regular, heuristic (self-correcting) basis in which changes in process are an ongoing part of program implementation.

Counselors must be not only engaged in the progression of student learning, they must also be able to demonstrate to administration and the public that they are responsible for positive results for students. Further, if counselors wish to show themselves to be indispensable, they must provide adequate evidence of those results in a high enough profile to impress a doubting audience. When students are asked to reflect on the impact of their school counselors in traditional programs, only occasionally does a student attribute academic, career, social, or personal success to the interventions of a school counselor. Considering the characteristics and training of school counselors, this is a disappointing outcome. Accountability means more than meeting the new demands of school politics; it is an absolute necessity for the stability of the school counseling community.

Teaming Traditionally, counselors have worked as individuals, attempting to meet all the needs of their assigned students. In the new approach, counselors and other student support professionals work as a team, utilizing the unique interests and skills of each team member to accomplish results. By legitimizing the inclusion of differentiated staffing, this model can lead to the possibility of career ladders and lattices. In addition, it includes development of student support teams in which counselors, school psychologists, school nurses, child welfare and attendance specialists, administrators, parents, and others work and plan together on a regular basis. Working closely as a team with others reduces territorial disputes, reduces duplication of efforts, and expands the program to address all students.

To achieve this outcome, school counselors must find ways to get out of the office, to interact and collaborate with a wide range of school and community personnel, and to develop new programs with partners to proactively and preventively reach a wider range of students. Using the results-based approach, partnerships have developed in which student support team members work closely with teachers, administrators, parents, community members, and others to provide more personalized approaches to a broader range of students, with greater success and measurable outcomes than were possible in the traditional model.

Inductive Planning Results-based student support programs are developed by counseling professionals using professional expertise and research on student needs as the source of student competencies to be addressed. Traditionally, counseling services have been designed based on needs assessments (i.e., asking teachers, students, parents, administrators, and community members what counselors should do) rather than asking questions about the competencies students themselves need to become successful.

Program Evaluation Evaluation of results-based student support programs is based on the number of students who demonstrate the competencies attained. In the past counseling services have been evaluated on the number of students receiving help, the number of services offered to students, and how the students felt about the services. Instead of this traditional method of counting and reporting how many things were accomplished by guidance, results-based programs draw a clear target before starting implementation and then are accountable for how many students attained the desired results.

Counselor Evaluation Counselors are no longer evaluated on teacher-normed criteria or in competition with their colleagues, with all counselors being measured by the same criteria (role and function statements). Counselors are now evaluated on their success in providing students with guidance-related competencies. A counselor's success in this system is based on the ability to create, select, and implement processes to attain the targeted student competencies. Counselors are encouraged to work as a team in collaboration with other student support professionals and other staff members in order to maximize the use of their individual skills and interests to reach all students.

Management/Leadership The administrator's role becomes one of reaching consensus on delineated results and plans, monitoring and appreciating processes, and coaching staff to attain new professional skills. This role replaces the traditional one of directing counselors' activities and judging their effectiveness based on criteria that are either elusive or developed for use with teachers. The actual program implementation is planned and managed by credentialed counselors, thereby relieving administrators of the need to act as a kind of department chairperson on a daily basis. Traditional organizational patterns often leave student support professionals torn between administrative needs and the directives of the vice principal in charge of guidance on one hand and student needs for learning, relating, and leading a balanced life on the other. When counselors manage their own programs, it is easier to address the needs of the system and the students to provide a balanced approach to reaching program goals.

Systems Orientation The new approach is proactive—that is, counselors must reach out to all students rather than waiting for students to request services. It is developmentally designed to address expected concerns and needs associated with normal stages of development. It is preventive: programs are planned systemically to anticipate issues and teaching skills that may be needed before a crisis demands emergency or remedial actions. This approach extends the skills of the counselor to include an educational component. Counselors no longer wait for the "teachable moment" and try, through crisis intervention, to help students solve their problems. Instead, they use a variety of delivery methods to teach students problem-solving skills. When a crisis occurs, the counselor guides the student through the steps of problem solving that they have already learned, so they can solve their own problems. Assuring that a counselor is available at all times becomes a major concern for crisis-oriented counseling services. In a results-based program, the student is less dependent on a counselor for a solution to every problem.

The Results-Based Programs Model Versus the Process-Based Services Model

We can enlarge on the differences between the results-based program approach to guidance and traditional guidance services by detailing their opposing philosophies in a range of areas. Although most educators are aware that few real-world programs align strictly with one perspective or the other, this list of key differences can help us to clearly distinguish between the models.

Services Versus Program

A *program* is a systemic effort to deliver specific student outcomes that have been identified as critical to student success. A program contains the elements of a system as consistent with systems theory and similar to other programs within a school, such as English, math, and social studies. *Services*, on the other hand, are designed to address the immediate concerns of students, staff and parents as they occur.

Helping Versus Teaching

In the guidance services model, the counselor helps students solve their problems. In the program model, the counselor teaches students problem-solving skills; the program focuses on ensuring that students gain knowledge, attitudes, and skills. In short, services *help* students, programs *teach* students. Once students learn problem-solving skills, it is assumed they will use those skills when problems occur. Students who come to a program-oriented counselor for help will be coached to use the skills they have already learned, not have their problems solved for them. A specific problem is seen as a "readiness" indicator that the time to cement problem-solving skills the student already learned has arrived.

What Counselors Will Do Versus What Students Will Learn

A *program* states what students will learn. *Services* identify what counselors will do to help students. In the program model, the question, "What do counselors do?" is changed to "What do students learn, and how are they different because of what they learn?" A frequent mistake of student support programs is to adopt a mission statement that indicates what the professionals will do (e.g., "encourage," "facilitate," etc.). Because a results-based program identifies the student as the primary client, the mission statement indicates what students will achieve through the program.

Who Determines Responsibilities: Administration Versus Counselor

In the traditional model, counselors operate from a role-and-function statement of duties and responsibilities defined by the administration. In contrast, a results-based program operates from the philosophy that the student support professional is the best judge of what will be successful in a specific situation. Activities are not predetermined; only the desired results are identified and agreed upon before a counselor plans the processes to be employed on a case-by-case basis to achieve the desired results in student competencies. In a results-based program, there is no attempt to control or regulate a counselor's time. The amount of time spent in the classroom, small groups, and individual sessions and with teachers, parents, community members, training tutors, and others is the counselor's choice. Each professional may use different activities to reach the same outcome based on the situation, resources, professional skills, student characteristics, and other variables. Each member of a student support team (counselor, school psychologist, nurse, social worker, other) will use his or her own repertoire of skills to ensure that students attain the desired result.

> In one case, a new counselor was given a role-and-function statement indicating that she should plan to see each student assigned to her a minimum of once each semester. Since the counselor had 550 students assigned to her, if she saw each student individually during class time, she was theoretically responsible for 1,100 classroom interruptions. That school had five counselors with comparable student caseloads and identical role-and-function statements. An outside consultant recommended that the counselor wait until the first all-school pep rally, go out to the middle of the athletic field, turn around 360 degrees and carefully "see" each and every student in attendance. Then she could go into her office and check off her list of duties, indicating that she had seen each student once that semester! The salient point was that absent any desired result when "seeing" the student, it doesn't matter when, where or how the task was completed. Only the completion of the task is counted, not the effectiveness.

Accountability: Process Versus Results

In theory, if processes are consistent in all situations, then one can logically expect a variable result. That is, if only one process, such as classroom presentations, is used, some students will learn and some will not. If the desired student result is guaranteed, then one must vary processes to ensure that all students attain the desired result. If only a percentage of the students reach the result after participating in a planned presentation, then new and different activities must be instituted to reach the remaining students who didn't achieve the first time. For those students, individual counseling, parent involvement, peer mentors, or other processes may be tried. In the results-based model, the counselor is accountable for the number of students who attain the indicated competency, not the number of students who listen to the presentation.

Student Educational Needs: Reacting Versus Planning Ahead

Traditional services frequently utilize counselor time and skills to fit students into the structure of the educational system. Counselors are called on to program students into classes on a master calendar that is predetermined. When there is a conflict, the counselor helps students choose among their limited options. Results-based programs focus instead on educational planning and utilize the counselor as an advocate to ensure that students have career plans, decision-making skills, and other competencies that allow them to identify their unique educational needs and provide information the counselors use in conference with administrators to plan appropriate courses and schedules. One system fits the student into the system; the other adapts the system to meet individual student needs.

Professional Responsibilities: Individual Assignments Versus Teamwork

Traditional services treat each group of professionals as separate entities. Individual counselors are assigned to a caseload of students based on one or more variables, which may include a set number of students whose last name begins with a letter in one section of the alphabet, or a class of students, or a specific focus usually based on categorical funding, or other criteria. The counselors' job is to provide the same services to all the students. School psychologists, social workers, nurses, and others work with specific students based on identified characteristics, such as learning difficulties, outside distracters, juvenile justice involvement, and health problems. Often the professionals in each of these disciplines report to different administrators, meet separately, and seldom discuss individual students with one another.

A student support team coordinates the efforts of a variety of professionals, responding to individual student needs in a cooperative manner. Individual students and groups of students are assessed by the team and appropriate interventions may occur through more than one discipline. All members of the team share a common purpose, mission, philosophy, and goal. There is mutual respect and collaboration among the groups. Staff members are assigned based on their area(s) of expertise rather than on their credentialing. Professionals may cross over in function if one person is more appropriately prepared than another to take on a task. One administrator monitors the entire student support program with all staff members who are part of the team.

For example, a team of counselors working together in a traditional program decided to try differential staffing and began by voicing their preferred assignment. One of the new counselors indicated that she preferred working with alienated, low-achieving students, especially gang-involved students. A more experienced counselor on the same team preferred to work with college-bound students. As they discussed a new way of dividing the caseload, the experienced counselor was concerned for his colleague and protested that it was unfair to give the new counselor the most difficult kids as her assignment. Her response was, "Why not? I'll have the fun, challenging kids and you'll get the boring kids." What a shame it would have been to deprive students of the skills of the experienced counselor, who had a reputation for advocating for students to get into the college of their choice, just because of a caseload mentality. Meanwhile, the new counselor turned out to have extraordinary talents in motivating the unmotivated students and providing a sense of belonging for alienated students. A traditional caseload approach would have deprived both sets of students. Through a series of decisions made by the counselors to most effectively meet student needs, this traditional program became a results-based program.

Deductive Versus Inductive Needs Assessment

Traditional programs are based on periodic needs assessments in which students, parents, teachers, and community members are queried about what they think students need. The responses are diverse and many times embody unattainable goals for students. If one accepts the definition of needs as "a gap in results" (Kaufman, 1972), then very few needs assessments identify actual needs; most identify "wants." This kind of *deductive* planning prioritizes immediate wants over research-based, data-based information from the discipline of counseling and other student support disciplines.

Results-based student support programs utilize an *inductive* planning process to establish program goals. That is, they rely on research findings, professional publications, and data-based information to inform decisions. The many years of study that go into preparing professionals are valued and utilized in the planning process. Wants may be considered, but the focus is on identifying needed student competencies and planning the program to ensure that all students are successful.

Program Evaluation: User Satisfaction Versus Student Results

Evaluation of the program is determined by the number of students who successfully attain the identified competencies before they graduate from the school. Traditional programs are often evaluated on a bean-counting basis—that is, counting the processes used (number of phone calls made to homes, number of classroom presentations, number of students visiting the career center, etc.) and the number of students involved in the processes. Another evaluation strategy for guidance services is the user satisfaction survey, which lets counselors know how popular or beneficial the service is to those who use the resource. It is assumed that the more students participate in the traditional program or receive services from the staff members, the more relevant and valuable the services.

In reality, it is possible for students to participate regularly and still fail to reach their goals and aspirations. When student success is the focus, staff members find themselves reaching out to others in the school community and the home to help students develop competencies to succeed. A student may not be participating regularly in the student support program because the counselor may have arranged a tutor, a church program, parents or grandparents, a job supervisor, or someone else to work with that student. The program is successful if the student learns what was planned.

Daily Counselor Activities: Reactive Versus Proactive

Traditional counselors spend much of their time in their offices, counseling individual students who are referred by themselves or others, doing paperwork related to school issues, going to meetings, or preparing materials to be handed out to students.

Results-based programs require counselors and other student support personnel to become proactive in their school communities. They spend time in classrooms making presentations, observing students, assisting the teacher in classroom behavior and learning skills, working with parents to encourage their presence in the school and classroom, and various other tasks that take them out of their offices and into the school community. Professionals in results-based programs find it necessary to make careful plans, set their own schedules, and determine timelines for attaining specific results.

Who Determines the Counseling Schedule: Administration Versus Counselor

Traditional counselors follow a predictable schedule based on the expectations delineated by the role-and-function statement and the job description they were given at the time they were hired. The school administrator or department chairperson directs and monitors the counselor's time. Counselors complain that they come to school each day and their day "happens to them." In these situations counselors find themselves acting as troubleshooters filling in for absent teachers; supervising cafeteria, restroom, and passing periods; following up on discipline referrals; planning for standardized testing; and similar stopgap tasks.

Results-based counselors, on the other hand, are encouraged to plan their own schedules, including a calendar that indicates when they plan to visit classrooms, conference with parents, hold individual conferences, implement group counseling, attend IEP meetings, and the like. Each member of the student support team is responsible for planning his or her own schedules, processes, and accountability for the outcome of their decisions in terms of student competencies.

Basis of Performance Evaluation: Complying with Administration Expectations Versus Achieving Results

In traditional programs, professionals are evaluated based on their compliance with district and school expectations defined by the role and function and/or administration. Administrators are assumed to understand what counselors, school psychologists, social workers, and other student support personnel should be doing with their time, and each evaluation is based on how well the individual completes the task compared with his or her colleagues who are charged with completing the same list of responsibilities.

Results-based professionals define their own jobs and are evaluated on the number of students who demonstrate the defined competencies. Individual contributions to the department, the school, the district, and the community comprise part of the evaluation, but the most important goal is student competency and academic achievement. Results-based professionals produce results that are commensurate with district and school goals as well as mission and accreditation requirements. They are an integral part of the staff and actively contribute to the students and to the entire school community.

Equal Opportunity for Students Versus Student Equity

Traditional programs proclaim *equal opportunity,* which translates to the pledge that any student who seeks time and help from a counselor or other student support team member will be seen and helped. Priorities are generally based on the "first person through the door" or most pressing crisis.

Results-based programs proclaim *equity,* or the pledge that every student will attain the specific competencies needed for success in school, life outside school, and the future. Even those students who do not choose guidance are included in this pledge. In the same way that students cannot opt out of required academic programs such as math, science, and English, they also cannot opt out of guidance. It is a program, available and required for every student. Success is not optional under this program; it is expected, it is required, and it is achieved.

■ ACTIVITY SET 1.1

Comparing Results-Based Programs and Process-Based Services

The following table summarizes the significant differences between managing student support programs from a results-based program position and the traditional services approach.

DIFFERENCES BETWEEN RESULTS-BASED PROGRAMS
AND PROCESS-BASED SERVICES

Results-Based Programs	Process-Based Services	How Do the Differences Between the Two Approaches Impact Schools on a Daily Basis?
1. Program elements are delineated and based on desired student outcomes.	**1.** Services are based on student demand and school needs.	
2. Focus is on the product (student results; i.e., what students learn).	**2.** Focus is on processes/activities (what counselors do).	
3. Contributions are determined by the individual counselor to get specific student results.	**3.** Contributions are determined by a preexisting role-and-function statement.	
4. Product is held constant; therefore, processes must be varied.	**4.** Process is held constant; therefore, product will vary.	
5. Focus is on individual students—how each student can/will learn competencies.	**5.** Focus is on the system—fitting the student into the school structure.	
6. Student support professionals work as a team to utilize each person's unique skills and interests to attain results for all students.	**6.** Student support professionals work as individuals and use their skills to try to meet all the needs of their assigned students.	
7. Program is inductively planned using data from current programs and from professional research to determine program goals.	**7.** Program is deductively planned based on what students, parents, and staff indicate they want counselors to do.	
8. Program is evaluated on the number of students demonstrating pre-set guidance competencies.	**8.** Program is evaluated on number of students participating in processes.	
9. Student support team members are proactive to assure that all students have guidance competencies.	**9.** Counselors primarily react to requests and referrals from students, parents, and administrators.	
10. Processes are frequently changed as new data on student competency attainment is generated. Processes are determined by the individual team members.	**10.** Counselors follow an established set of processes, based on a role-and-function statement defined by the school administration.	
11. Personnel evaluations are based on the individual's contributions and ability to produce student results.	**11.** Personnel evaluations are based on established expectations, defined by administration for all counselors.	
Equity: All students will attain specified competencies.	*Equal opportunity:* Students can choose.	

■ **ACTIVITY SET 1.1 (CONTINUED)**

Discuss in a small group or write your response to the following questions:

1. What instigated the initial guidance efforts in schools?

2. What current forces are propelling the development of results-based student support programs?

■ REFLECTION

Please post your reflections on the evolution of the results-based student support model of school counseling.

_____

_____

_____

_____

■ SUMMARY

The time for change in the structure of guidance programs has arrived if guidance is to escape from the add-on syndrome and the deficiencies of a reactive approach. Results-based student support programs offer an alternative to existing programs by making the paradigm shift to guaranteed student results. The new approach focuses on the student as the primary client, not on the services being provided. By clearly identifying individual accountability for specific students results, counselors are encouraged to break out of established boundaries, become more creative, and involve others in the process. Involving others also provides a way to share skills, build a caring community, and expand the resources available to help students.

CHAPTER TWO

Elements of a Results-Based Student Support Program

Upon completion of this chapter and its activities, you should be able to demonstrate the following competencies:

- **Understand the 12 elements in the results-based program and know how the elements fit together to form a comprehensive system.**

- **Recognize the function and purpose of each element.**

■ *Introduction*

The results-based student support program (Johnson & Johnson, 1991) consists of a system of interrelated and interdependent elements. It demonstrates the congruence between student support programs and the school and district's mission, philosophy, curriculum, and other programs. The circular model in Figure 2.1 demonstrates the importance of a flow of elements: from the delineation of results, which are defined through the first five elements, to the processes that explain the means used to reach the results. Although programs do not require every element to be in place, for evaluation purposes the program must clearly stipulate the student results as identified in the mission, philosophy, goals, and glossary. The system can be entered at any point of the circle, but its strength derives from the fact that when any element is changed, the entire system changes to accommodate the new perspective. Nothing is rigid; the system is fluid and in a constant state of flux. It is also important to remember, however, that no one element can stand alone.

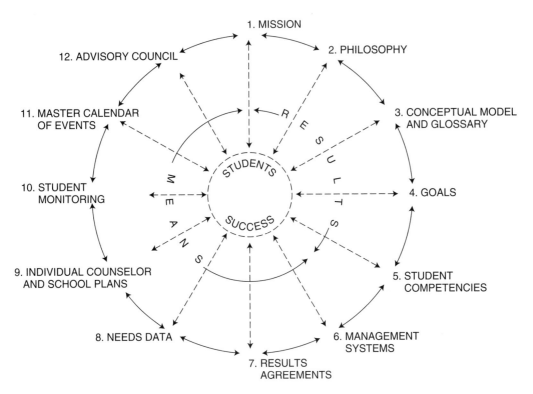

FIGURE 2.1

Copyright © 1981 C. D. Johnson and S. K. Johnson.

■ *Results Elements*

The elements that define the results of the program are:

1. *Mission (Vision, Purpose)* These statements define the intention of the guidance and/or student support program. They provide direction for all student goals and program activities by specifying the desired long-range (5+ years) results for *all* students. The desired long-range impact of the student support program must directly link with the statement of purpose, vision, or mission of the board of education and administration. The mission statement is the vehicle for clarifying the relationship between the educational system and the student support program.

As the element that defines what the student support program contributes to the educational program, the mission statement provides the foundation for building a student support team. When all student support professionals share the same vision and mission, it is a reasonable consequence that working together will increase the chances of reaching the target. Including all professional support groups within a school or district in developing the mission statement ensures that the unique perspectives and direction of each group is represented and that all groups have equal input and, thus, equal responsibility to help fulfill the program's intent.

2. *Philosophy* The philosophy is an articulated set of guiding principles that are used in the development, implementation, management, and evaluation of the program. The principles (usually a set of "we agree" statements) address all students, focus on prevention, specify the management system, indicate how counselors will maintain their professional competencies, and indicate the ethical guidelines to be followed by all counselors. Agreeing on the philosophy allows teams to form without having to renegotiate how individuals will work together and toward what end. In essence, the philosophy states, "This is what we believe about student support programs, this is how we will work together to reach our goals, these are our shared responsibilities, and this is how we will evaluate our work together."

3. *Glossary* The glossary ensures clarity of all terms included in the program description. It is imperative that guidance and counseling specialists make their specialized language accessible so that others can work comfortably with them as team members. The glossary is a definition of terms, written at a basic reading level, to ensure that team members, administrators, students, parents, and community members clearly understand all aspects of the program and therefore can work in concert to ensure student success. The glossary also identifies the models and theories that are used within the program (e.g., the definition of *decision making* in the glossary identifies the specific model or theory and elements of decision making that are used in program activities). The terms identified in the glossary form the basis of what will be evaluated. Evaluation of the program's success is based on measurement of elements and sub-elements as they are defined in the glossary (Johnson & Whitfield, 1991). It is almost impossible to evaluate anything that does not have a single clear definition that is accepted by everyone involved in the process. (See Appendix A for a sample glossary.)

4. *Goals* Goals are an extension of the statement of mission (purpose) and define the specific desired results to be achieved by the time a student leaves the school system. They are stated in terms of the knowledge, attitudes, and skills the student needs to become successful in higher education, advanced training, work, and/or other meaningful endeavors in the adult world. The goals are written in global terms for each of the domains identified in the program model; they usually include an educational or academic goal, a career or occupational goal, a social goal, and a personal goal (addressing leisure and wellness).

5. *Competencies* Competencies consist of developed proficiencies that are observable, transferable from a learning situation to a real-life situation, and directly aligned to a guidance goal. Student support professionals, students, parents, and staff use competencies as indicators to measure whether students are moving toward the stated goals. Competencies are defined by grade level (Appendix B). For example, study skills may be a goal within the education domain but vary depending upon the grade level; a ninth grader needs to learn different study skills than a third grader even though both need to know how to study effectively at their own level. Sometimes competencies are grouped into benchmarks at key transitional grade levels (Appendix C) that can be assessed collectively to determine progress toward a specific goal.

The following elements define how the program is implemented. They are the means.

6. *Management system (data flow schedule)* The management system deals with the allocation of resources to best address specified goals. It is also the process by which program and individual accountability for results is established. It identifies those responsible for students' acquisition of predetermined competencies, what data will be generated, how the data will be collected, and when the data will be submitted to the administrator. The management system also makes clear the division between student results, for which student support professionals assume accountability, and duties assigned by the administrator. The management system also identifies the reciprocal function of the administrator responsible for the student support program and each student support team member. The management system facilitates communication and the flow of data that are vital to making necessary mid-course corrections in program plans.

7. *Results agreements* These are responsibility statements made by each student support team member, specifying the results for which she or he has chosen to be accountable. The results are expressed in terms of the competencies students will achieve, are closely linked to the program goals, and include a separate section for all assigned duties. Additional results are specified for parents, staff, and self-improvement. The administrator responsible for the student support program will be active in reviewing, negotiating, and arriving at consensus on the results agreements. A district director of student support programs (or comparable position) audits the results agreements to assure that the assigned duties are not disproportionate to similar responsibilities expected of all teachers. Once the results agreement is accepted, the counselor is accountable for achievement of the agreed-upon student results and is responsible for carrying out the identified processes for assigned duties.

8. *Needs data* Needs identify the gap between the desired results and results currently being achieved. They are directly related to the goals and student competencies defined for the program. This model of student support is an inductively planned system that uses needs assessment to validate the program goals and to indicate priorities within the program parameters. Inductive needs assessments allow the professional staff to use their expertise and the structure provided by a conceptual model to design a comprehensive program to meet the needs of all students. Needs data are used to complete a competency assessment of students and to determine the amount and type of resources and effort needed to assist all students in achieving the expected level of proficiency.

9. *Results plans* Plans completed by individual team members indicate how results will be achieved. These plans contain the competency (specific knowledge, skill, or attitude) to be achieved, the criteria for success, who does what, where and when the process will be done, the activities and resources to be used, and how the evaluation will be done. The plans are always flexible and can be changed as data are collected and reflected upon. The underlying assumption is that if a process turns out to be less successful than projected, it may be best to change processes midstream in order to achieve the maximum results. Team members are urged to discontinue ineffective processes as soon as it is clear that results are not forthcoming, even if the process works for others. Individual professionals must assume responsibility for their own processes and their success or lack of success in attaining student results. Administrators must be willing to accept flexible processes as part of the results-based philosophy.

10. *Monitoring system* This system ensures that each student acquires the specified competencies. It is designed to communicate to students and parents the individual student's progress in attaining guidance-related goals. The process includes a responsible adult (parent, teacher, boss, neighbor, etc.) who observes or measures demonstrations of competency and records verification on a form or student folder. Many schools choose to use a paper or computer-generated guidance portfolio (Appendix F) to monitor student progress and encourage students to maintain and update a record of the specific competencies they have attained. Monitoring of academic achievement must be completed at regular times within each school term and include interventions when students fall below expectations. Schools that include regular and consistent monitoring of academic achievement show significant improvement in grades and test scores. Of greatest importance is the shared responsibility by student, parent, and teacher for monitoring the student's progress, especially in the area of academic achievement, and to institute interventions when the level of achievement is unacceptable.

11. *Master calendar of events* A calendar of student support events is published to communicate the what, when, and where of program activities to students, teachers, parents, administrators, and community members. This calendar serves as a communication vehicle and increases the program's visibility in the school, the district, and the community. It is important to distribute the calendar widely among teachers so that they are aware of the programs available to their students to help improve grades (such as study skills. test-taking skills, organizational skills, etc.) and among parents so that they and their children can attend relevant functions (including college and career fairs, financial aid workshops, etc.). Distribution within the community ensures that others are also aware of the contributions made by student support programs to the community and its children.

12. *Advisory council* The advisory council is an ongoing body of individuals that includes representation of all groups affected by the program (i.e., parents, teachers, student support staff, administration, local community groups, and students when appropriate). The purpose of the council is to review student support program results and recommend priorities to the appropriate administrative body. When the advisory council is formed and managed efficiently, the members can become the most vocal advocates for the student support program. Often the advisory council members volunteer or are invited to appear before the school board to advocate for changes, such as an increase in staff, materials, space, and funding. It is always more effective to have others speak in support of the program than to have counselors or other student support professionals trying to justify the program's needs.

■ REFLECTION

Express your thoughts about the elements of a results-based student support program.

_____

_____

_____

_____

_____

■ SUMMARY

The results-based student support model is a systems approach for putting together a comprehensive program that reaches all students. In essence, "the discipline of systems thinking lies in a shift of mind: seeing interrelationships rather than linear cause-effect chains and seeing processes of change rather than snapshots" (Senge, 1990). Although each element is developed for a single purpose, together all of the elements form a complete system that defines the results as well as the system means to reach the results. However, the system does not dictate how individual districts, schools, and professionals plan and implement curriculum, spend their time, allocate resources, or deliver professional services. It holds the results constant but allows flexibility and creativity within the processes.

PART TWO

Results

CHAPTER THREE

Establishing the Mission

Upon completion of this chapter and its activities, you should be able to demonstrate the following competencies:

- **Recognize the importance of a mission statement and how it guides the student support program**

- **Understand how the mission statement links the student support program with the mission of education locally and nationally**

- **Understand how the mission delineates the vision, purpose, long-range goals, and underlying beliefs about students**

- **Develop an effective mission statement**

■ *Introduction*

The *mission statement* lays the foundation for building a comprehensive results-based student support program. It provides the context for the issues and decisions that are made on a regular basis as well as a framework for communicating to students, parents, and other educators what we want our students to achieve and become. The ideas generated within the mission must be the guide for the daily activities of the program. If the mission is tucked away and forgotten, the program can easily become a reactive, crisis-oriented service called on only to meet immediate needs. The student support mission must also directly link with the educational mission of the nation, the state, the district and the school.

■ *The Mission Statement*

The mission statement is the first element that must be developed in a results-based program. It is essential to each of the subsequent elements and, in the end, becomes the measure by which the entire program is judged. In working through the program step by step, it becomes evident that the strength and solidity of the mission sustains the program, including the determination of results, processes, and evaluation. When aspects of the program become muddled or unclear during the process of program development, the mission statement shines a light on the purpose, direction, meaning, and commitment and keeps the process moving forward.

What Is the Mission Statement?

The mission statement states the purpose of the program, lays down the vision, and specifies the long-range goals that will guide the program's directions. It provides the target for the energy and commitment of the professional staff members.

What Does the Mission Statement Contribute to the Program?

The mission statement

- Confirms that the student is the primary client.
- Declares the program's intentions.
- Focuses on the program's primary purpose.
- Defines the commitment to a common purpose.
- Clarifies the beliefs and philosophy underlying the program.
- Provides a communication tool to ensure clarity in decision making.
- Establishes the same goals for all student support professionals (mission, purpose, unity not uniformity, oneness not sameness).

What Questions Does the Mission Statement Answer?

The mission statement answers three key questions:

1. *What is the purpose?* The primary purpose is to ensure that all students gain the competencies necessary to become successful, productive citizens in their schools, families, and communities.
2. *Who is the client?* The student is the primary client.
3. *What does the school community value?* Students as well as parents and educators agree that academic achievement, career development, positive relationships with others, and a healthy and balanced personal lifestyle are the goals for student success.

Where Does the Mission Fit in a Program?

The mission is developed at the beginning of a program, a curriculum, a business plan, or a personal plan. It is the basis for the rest of the elements of the program. On the basis of the mission, plans are derived, outcomes are made visible, and team members become aware of both program and individual accountability. The mission identifies the same target for everyone.

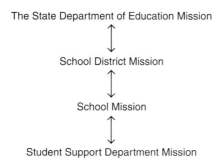

■ **FIGURE 3.1** *Hierarchy of Linkages*

Linkages

Every educational organization, including the state department of education, the school district, the individual school, school departments, and many individual educators all have their own mission. These mission statements are linked together by same or similar intention, results, and accountability. As illustrated in Figure 3.1, the missions of related (educational) organizations must be linked to ensure that all educators operate within the same parameters.

The focus of linkages narrow as each level seeks to define the unique contributions of the individuals represented at that level. For example, when the state department mission defines academic achievement as the primary focus, the school district must echo that goal and so must the school and the student support program. It is unlikely that a program not in alignment with the primary focus of the nation, the state, the district, and the school will be maintained, especially when budgets are cut and layoffs imminent. If a district identifies academic achievement as the primary focus, the school will define its own responsibility and each department will assume a part of the academic mission. Student support is a part of the whole system, and as a part must define what segment of the total responsibility will be accepted by the student support staff. In a climate focused on achievement, a program designed to address mental health issues is in danger of cuts no matter how admirable the intent or how important the results.

An old adage states, "When you work for Ford, you build Fords. You don't build Chevrolets." Likewise, when the education system establishes the mission, departments within the system must support that mission. If the mission is not acceptable to a department, then it is seen as an appendage, not part of the mainstream. Counselors and other support personnel can lobby for other considerations, present data, and advocate for individual students, but when the bottom line is determined, only those professionals and departments aligned with the stated mission will be supported. Unfortunately, although it is viable for business, this protocol often deprives students of valuable experiences, such as vocational programs and development of hobbies. In response to these losses within educational systems, collaboration with community resources becomes a high priority for comprehensive student support programs. Much of the support must come from community resources when school resources fall short.

Some Additional Questions and Answers

Understanding why a mission is critical and how it becomes an integral and visible part of the program lays the foundation for taking the task of establishing a mission seriously.

Why Does the Student Support Program Need a Separate Statement of Mission? Student support programs are accountable for specific program results that are different from, but related to, other curricula. Guidance has a set of standards issued by the American School Counselors Association (Campbell & Dahir, 1997) to help local school counselor teams developing their own standards. A separate mission promotes program and personnel visibility. It is important to have a common set of beliefs to avoid becoming distracted by the insignificant and forgetting the agreed-upon outcomes. Here the mission serves as a reference point, a reminder.

How Do Teachers, Administrators, Students, and Parents Become Aware of the Student Support Team Mission Statement? Other educators within the school need to know that the student support team has developed and believes in its mission statement. The statement establishes that the student support program is accountable for student results just like other educational programs. Teams should make copies of the mission statement along with their philosophy, goals, and desired student competencies on a poster-sized printout and post them in every classroom, the guidance office, the parent center, and local community and business organizations.

■ **ACTIVITY SET 3.1**

Develop a Mission Statement

The purpose of this activity is to produce a mission statement that meets the criteria used in the results-based program. Please understand that the steps given here are only guides; you might choose to develop the mission in a different way. Each student or team of students develops a mission statement for the student support program at a specific school, district, or organization. The content of the statement will meet the following criteria:

1. Written with the student as the primary client.

2. Written for all students.

3. Indicates the content and competencies to be learned.

4. Shows linkages between the statement of mission or purpose and those of the school, school district, and state department of education.

5. Indicates the long-range (5–10 years after graduation) results (outcomes) desired for all students.

A. Evaluation of sample mission statements as student teams. Discuss the following sample statements and identify what should be included and/or excluded in each.

Example 1

State Department of Education Mission Statement

The mission of the Utopia Department of Education is to provide equal access to a quality education for every student and to promote world-class standards in every school.

1. Complete the following statements about the sample:

   a. The primary client is _____.

   b. The population for which it is written is _____.

   c. The content is _____.

   d. Linkage evidence is _____.

   e. Long-range results/outcomes are_____.

2. List the words/terminology in this mission statement that you think should be in the glossary:

   _____ _____ _____

   _____ _____ _____

   _____ _____ _____

District Board of Education Mission Statement

The Utopia Unified School District exists to develop responsible, lifelong learners capable of molding the future.

1. Complete the following statements about the sample:

   a. The primary client is _____.

   b. The population for which it is written is _____.

   c. The content is _____.

   d. Linkage evidence is _____.

   e. Long-range results/outcomes are_____.

2. List the words/terminology you think should be in the glossary:

   _____ _____ _____

   _____ _____ _____

   _____ _____ _____

Local School Mission Statement

Utopia Middle School provides each student with a diverse education in a safe, supportive environment that promotes self-discipline, motivation, and excellence in learning to ensure that students become independent and self-sufficient adults who will succeed and contribute responsibly in a global community.

1. Complete the following statements about the sample:

   a. The primary client is _____.

   b. The population for which it is written is _____.

   c. The content is _____.

   d. Linkage evidence is _____.

   e. Long-range results/outcomes are_____.

2. List the words/terminology you think should be in the glossary:

_____   _____   _____

_____   _____   _____

_____   _____   _____

Student Support Program Mission

The mission of the student support program is to ensure that all students acquire the skills in learning, working, relating to others, and making healthy lifestyle choices needed to become independent and self-sufficient adults in a global community.

1. Complete the following statements about the sample:

   a. The primary client is _____.

   b. The population for which it is written is _____.

   c. The content is _____.

   d Linkage evidence is _____.

   e. Long-range results/outcomes are_____.

2. List the words/terminology you think that should be in the glossary:

_____   _____   _____

_____   _____   _____

_____   _____   _____

Example 2

District Board of Education Mission Statement

The mission of the Utopia public schools is to prepare students for a lifetime of learning and productive, meaningful participation in a complex, changing world.

1. Complete the following statements about the sample:

   a. The primary client is _____.

   b. The population for which it is written is _____.

   c. The content is _____.

   d. Linkage evidence is _____.

   e. Long-range results/outcomes are _____.

2. List the words/terminology you think that should be in the glossary:

_____   _____   _____

_____   _____   _____

_____   _____   _____

Local School Mission Statement

The mission of Utopia High School is to provide a comprehensive educational experience for each student to attain quality academic preparation, problem-solving skills, citizenship skills, and respect for self and others in a diverse, complex world.

1. Complete the following statements about the sample:

   a. The primary client is _____.

   b. The population for which it is written is _____.

   c. The content is _____.

   d. Linkage evidence is _____.

   e. Long-range results/outcomes are _____.

  2. List the words/terminology you think should be in the glossary:

_____ _____ _____

_____ _____ _____

_____ _____ _____

Student Support Mission Statement

The student support program has been developed to ensure that each student in Utopia High School will acquire necessary competencies (knowledge, skills, attitudes) in educational planning, career planning, personal and social development in preparation for meaningful participation in a complex, changing world.

  1. Complete the following statements about the sample:

   a. The primary client is _____.

   b. The population for which it is written is _____.

   c. The content is _____.

   d. Linkage evidence is _____.

   e. Long-range results/outcomes are _____.

  2. List the words/terminology you think should be in the glossary:

_____ _____ _____

_____ _____ _____

_____ _____ _____

B. Mission Statement. You will now develop a mission statement for an actual or imagined school, school district, or other educational organization. The first activity is to choose words or statements that fulfill the criteria requirements. Please complete the requested information:

  1. The primary client is _____.

  2. The population for which it is written is _____.

  3. The content is _____.

  4. Linkage evidence is _____.

  5. Long-range results/outcomes are _____.

Using the information generated here, write your completed statement of mission.

_____

_____

_____

_____

_____

_____

_____

_____

_____

_____

Please list all the words you believe should be defined for others to understand your program mission. If possible, define them here (or you may complete the task at a later date).

_____ _____ _____

_____ _____ _____

_____ _____ _____

_____ _____ _____

_____ _____ _____

C. Upon completion of your mission statement. Ask a colleague to check your responses. If you are in a group, request another member to check for the following:

1. Are all words that might have more than one understanding underlined for inclusion in the glossary?

2. Are identified results accomplishments that remain appropriate for several (5–10) years after graduation rather than skills expected at time of graduation?

3. Are specific guidance-related results identified? For example, ensuring that all students are lifelong learners is an appropriate mission for the district or school, but the specific contribution of the student support program may be to ensure that each student gains appropriate skills in becoming an effective learner. These include study skills, test-taking skills, and knowledge of one's unique learning style.

4. Does the student support mission statement have a direct link with the district and school mission? Are there parallel words or phrases within all three (district, school, and student support program) mission statements?

5. Is the student support mission concrete enough to be measured if students are assessed 10 years after graduation?

If your colleague or another team judges your mission statement to be weak, please discuss it again and decide if you wish to change the statement in order to clarify it to all stakeholders. Polish the statement and identify additional words or terms that should be part of the glossary.

(Be careful of words such as *enable, facilitate, help,* and *assist.* These describe what staff members do, not what the students learn. The program's mission is not to provide services; it is to ensure student success.)

■ REFLECTION

Please reflect on the activity you have just finished, indicating what you think is usable, what you think isn't, and why. What importance does a mission statement have for your continuing exploration of student support programs? Reflect on the process and on the beliefs, values, and commitment necessary to provide a results-based program that addresses the needs of each student.

_____

_____

_____

_____

_____

_____

_____

■ SUMMARY

In this chapter we discussed how school-based programs must align their mission with those of the district and state education systems and have examined how the mission sets the direction for future developments. In this section you have had the opportunity to acquire knowledge and skills in developing the mission statement for a results-based student support program. After reaching consensus on the values that will guide the program's direction, it is necessary to examine and agree upon beliefs that set the boundaries for implementation. Because a variety of disciplines participate in a student support team, the concept of boundaries is needed to ensure respect for the different skills, training, and responsibilities within the program. Clarity of boundaries and shared commitment becomes essential to smooth implementation and a collaborative working relationship. The guiding principles of the program are established through a philosophy reflecting the collective personal and professional priorities of team members. The next step in developing a results-based student support program is preparing a program philosophy statement.

CHAPTER FOUR

Establishing the Philosophy

Upon completion of this chapter and its activities, you should be able to demonstrate the following competencies:

- **Understand the role of the program philosophy in determining how the program will operate, who will manage the activities, who will be involved, and what professional ethics and guidelines will be used to maintain program and individual ethics**

- **Use consensus to develop a program philosophy**

- **Use data from individuals to recognize strengths and potential areas of contribution to students**

■ *Introduction*

Once a mission statement has been accepted, the next step is developing an agreed-upon *philosophy* or set of "we agree" statements that will act as the guiding principles for the work ahead. In his book, *The Structure of Scientific Revolutions* (1970), Kuhn states: "No single theory will ever give us a perfect or all purpose point of view" (p. 5). In much the same way, there is no perfect philosophy of student support; each program crafts a philosophy that reflects the individuals who make up the team and identifies how they will work together to define and achieve success.

By completing the activities in this chapter, you will develop or revisit your worldview and through consensus participate in developing a school-based philosophy that addresses the major issues of who benefits from the student support program, how the program is developed, who will manage the activities, who will evaluate the results, and what ethical mandates will be followed. The activities also offer an opportunity to learn more about others' personal and professional philosophies.

■ *Definition of Terms*

In order to communicate as a team, it is necessary to ascertain that all members share a common understanding of the terms used within the program.

Philosophy

The *philosophy* is a set of guiding principles agreed upon and followed by the individuals implementing a student support program. It is important that all personnel involved in managing and implementing the program achieve consensus on each principle or "we agree" statement. Consensus does not mean that each participant must agree completely with each principle; it means that all can live with the statements being proposed.

Principles

For professional counselors and other support personnel, certain areas of a guiding philosophy are covered by principles or beliefs. These are derived in part from the personal convictions and professional expectations of the participating individuals.

Program Philosophy

The program philosophy is a

- Set of principles that guide professional contributions.
- Set of beliefs that motivate program innovations.
- Statement of conduct for professional actions.
- Set of values that is visible to all.
- Source of collective power.

What does the philosophy provide?

- Sources of power to develop a specific program
- Authority to implement the program
- A sense of security
- Access to all student support resources
- Authority to define the program's decision processes
- Direction for use of effective organizational structures, rules, and regulations
- Permission to moderate professional boundaries within certification limitations
- Emphasis on a team learning community
- A set of professional behaviors and the determination to achieve the results delineated in the mission

■ **ACTIVITY SET 4.1**
Developing a Program Philosophy

This activity clarifies the process of writing a program philosophy statement. Because your personal philosophy will infuse meaning and heart into the program statements, we start there.

Personal Philosophy or Worldview

As a graduate student, you may have been asked to develop and write your own personal philosophy of counseling. A comprehensive philosophic framework is also called a *worldview*. Now is a good time to revisit this philosophy or worldview, reevaluate it, and compare it to the philosophies of your colleagues or other members of the student support team. If you have not already written your own philosophy, try sitting down and writing what you believe about the world, about community, about education, and about school counseling before starting the formal exercise in which you will write a cohesive philosophy for your school-based student support program.

A. Your answers to the following seven questions can be used as a guide to develop a worldview.

1. Who are we? Who am I? *(These questions address the heart of your reasons for wanting to be a counselor, school psychologist, school social worker, etc.)*

_____

_____

_____

_____

_____

2. Why is the world the way it is? How do I fit into that world? *(For many, the world is their own community or their school community. In today's world, a global perspective is essential for a number of reasons, including understanding our diverse populations, the economy, the job market, and career planning parameters; understanding youth culture, music, idols, etc.)*

_____

_____

_____

_____

_____

3. Where are we going? What are the possibilities and alternatives? Which of the different alternatives should we promote and which should we avoid? (*Our students are the adults and leaders of the future. The guidance we provide can establish a life direction for students. We should not be making decisions for ourselves or others without careful consideration of all possible alternatives.*)

_____

_____

_____

_____

4. What ethic or system of rules guides my decisions? (*Professional organizations work diligently to bring together the best thinkers in a field to craft ethical standards. However, even if we accept the standards developed in our discipline, it is important to find ways to incorporate our own ethics, values, and beliefs into our decisions.*)

_____

_____

_____

_____

5. How should we act? What is my plan of action? (Professing a worldview but leaving it within the realm of idealism without taking action to support one's beliefs is unconscionable. Anticipating how we might act and react in specific situations makes a specific worldview more comprehensive.)

_____

_____

_____

_____

_____

6. How do I construct my model of a worldview? How do I see the world, family and community groups, work, and individual worth? (*Format and style differ for every individual. Some use metaphors to frame their ideas; others work from a philosophical or religious viewpoint; still others use a list of seemingly unrelated statements that highlight areas of most importance to them. There is no right way, only your way.*)

_____

_____

_____

_____

7. What building blocks (theories, models, concepts, values, disciplines, and guidelines) are important in the development of my worldview? (*Trust yourself and trust the process. Your worldview can and will change over time as you incorporate new experiences and new insights along the way. This is no one-time exercise; it is an evolving expression of self.*)

_____

_____

_____

_____

B. Using your answers to the previous seven questions as a guide, write your personal philosophy or worldview.

_____

_____

_____

_____

_____

_____

_____

_____

_____

_____

_____

_____

_____

_____

_____

_____

C. Once you have reread your philosophy and compared it with those written by other class members, you will develop a philosophical statement or a set of 'we agree' statements that would be acceptable within a given school environment and also expresses your personal beliefs. This philosophy provides a framework that ties everything together as a guide to understanding society, the world, education and the position of guidance within education. It will be used in making critical decisions that will shape students' futures. The statement synthesizes the wisdom gathered through different scientific disciplines, personal philosophies, and counseling theories. Rather than focusing on small sections of reality, the philosophy provides an overview of the whole. In particular, this element helps to understand, and therefore cope with, complexity and change.

_____

_____

_____

_____

_____

_____

_____

_____

_____

_____

_____

_____

■ **ACTIVITY SET 4.2**

Develop the Philosophy for the Student Support Program

Form a group with others in the class to consider possible content and help one another to develop a tentative philosophy statement and explore as a group the complex issues from many points of view. At times "we become trapped in the theater of our own thoughts" (Senge, 1990, 231). Dialogue helps reveal the lack of clarity in individual thinking and is productive when the following three conditions are met:

1. All participants suspend their assumptions in order to hear others.

2. All participants regard one another as colleagues with valuable input.

3. A facilitator is present to hold the context of dialogue. (Senge, 1990, pp. 241–243)

A. After appointing a leader/facilitator, discuss the following criteria for an effective statement of philosophy. A philosophy for student support programs should:

1. Address all students.

2. Focus on primary prevention and student development.

3. Identify persons to be involved in the delivery or program activities.

4. Specify who will plan and who will manage the program.

5. Identify the management system to be used.

6. Define how the program will be evaluated and by whom.

7. Specify who will be responsible for monitoring students' academic, career, and personal/social development.

8. Specify how and when the team members will update and acquire new professional competencies; include ethical guidelines or standards.

B. Please review the following two examples and determine if they include the criteria delineated under item A. If not, indicate what would change.

Example 1

The counselors in Utopia public schools believe that

1. All students have the right to be served by the student support program.

2. The student support program is based on stated *goals** and delineated *student competencies.*

3. The student support program is consistent with *expected developmental stages* of learning.

4. *Student support program activities* are planned and coordinated by the counseling staff.

5. Student support program activities are *implemented* at each school by the counselors, school psychologists, social workers, child welfare and attendance

*Words and phrases that are italicized are examples of words to be specifically defined in your program glossary.

professionals, paraprofessionals, speech therapists, administrators, teachers, students, other staff, parents, and *community members* (as appropriate).

6. The student support program is *managed* by credentialed student support professionals.

7. Student support program managers present *evidence* of goal attainment at prespecified intervals during the school year.

8. All students

   - Have *access* to a school staff member to discuss personal concerns.

   - Have access to information about occupational and educational planning.

   - Have the *right to assistance* in identifying their self-characteristics.

   - Have the opportunity to make choices within the constraints of the educational system.

9. Students and staff are encouraged to recognize and appreciate the unique contributions, rights, responsibilities, and self-esteem of others.

10. Student support program services are available to local community members as resources allow.

11. Each student and parent is responsible for *monitoring* the student's educational progress with the assistance of school personnel.

12. An ongoing program of counselor *competency renewal* is necessary to maintain a quality student support program.

13. The professional mandates and guidelines proposed by the American School Counselor Association shall constitute *minimal standards* for the student support program.

Example 2

All counselors in Utopia public schools agree that

- The student support program is a *right* and shall serve all students in grades K–12.

- The student support program shall be evaluated on stated goals and related student competencies.

- The student support program shall be consistent with expected developmental stages of learning.

- Student support program activities will involve the *entire school community.*

- Student support program activities shall be determined and planned by the local school counseling staff *in consultation with* other representatives of the school community.

- The student support program shall be managed by state credentialed or licensed counselors using *participatory management* concepts and practices.

- Students shall have access to a counselor with whom they may discuss their concerns.

- Each student shall have individual freedom and responsibility of choices within the *constraints* of the local, county, and state educational systems.

- School personnel, students, and parents/guardians are responsible for monitoring the student's progress in school.

- A mandatory ongoing program of counselor competency renewal (training and retraining) is necessary to maintain a quality student support program. Competency renewal is a shared responsibility of the student support professionals, administrators, and the coordinator of the student support program.

- The professional mandates and ethical guidelines proposed by the American School Counselor Association are the basis of the standards for the student support program.

C. With another individual or in a group, develop a set of philosophy statements for a student support program at a specific school/work situation. Use the suggested criteria as a guide. Also use a consensus process to build the philosophy.

_____

_____

_____

_____

_____

_____

_____

_____

_____

_____

_____

_____

_____

_____

_____

_____

_____

_____

_____

_____

_____

_____

_____

D. List words and phrases used in the program philosophy that should be included in a glossary of terms.

_____   _____   _____

_____   _____   _____

_____   _____   _____

E. Upon completion of the program philosophy, ask another class member outside your own group to check for the following:

1. Are the language and meaning of terms clear (if not, are the words identified for inclusion in the glossary)? For example, terms such as *manager, administrator, implementer,* and *planner* may have different connotations to different people on the team.

Comments:_____

_____

_____

_____

_____

_____

2. Is there consistency in philosophy between statements—that is, are all statements compatible with participative management (if that is the identified management system)?

    Comments: _____

    _____

    _____

    _____

    _____

3. Is it clear who is responsible for each program function, such as developing the program, planning activities, monitoring student progress, implementing the program, program administration, and evaluation?

    Comments: _____

    _____

    _____

    _____

    _____

4. Are the roles of nonguidance participants (e.g., parents, staff, community members, students, district and school administrators) clear?

    Comments: _____

    _____

    _____

    _____

    _____

5. Are there questions that might occur to someone outside your team upon first reading the philosophy? Can these potential questions be addressed ahead of time?

Comments:_____

_____

_____

_____

_____

_____

■ REFLECTION

Reflect on your experiences in developing your worldview and a school-based program philosophy.

_____

_____

_____

_____

_____

_____

_____

■ SUMMARY

In this section you have had an opportunity to develop competencies in writing your worldview and in using your identified beliefs to establish a student support program philosophy through consensus with other members. You had opportunities to experience the programmatic and personal power of establishing a common philosophy. In the next section, you will learn about the conceptual model for student support programs.

CHAPTER FIVE

Using the Conceptual Model and Building a Glossary

Upon completion of this chapter and its activities, you should be able to demonstrate the following competencies:

- **Describe the use of the conceptual model presented in this chapter as a guide in developing a comprehensive and unique program**

- **Understand that every model sets limitations on what results are to be included and excluded**

- **Understand the importance of the glossary, which provides a vehicle for communication among all stakeholders**

- **Know how to build a glossary from authoritative sources**

■ *Introduction*

A *conceptual model* serves as a framework for the development of ideas within a discipline. The conceptual model provided here was developed early in the history of the guidance field and is still being used as a guide to the parameters of a comprehensive student support program. It is of

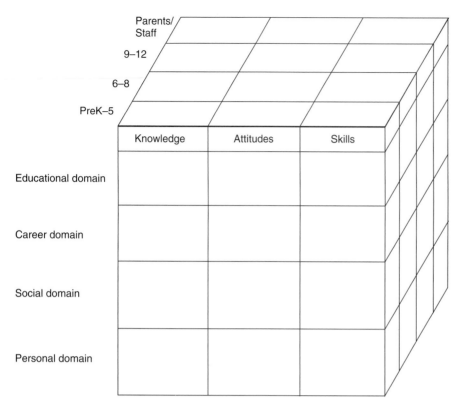

■ **FIGURE 5.1**
Adapted from Wellman National Study of Guidance Taxonomy of Objectives (1962).

limited use without clear definitions of each term and each domain. In using educational terminology, it is important to make sure that the glossary is written in clear, simple language so that readers from a variety of backgrounds can understand what is meant. In the second part of this chapter, we will discuss how to identify and record terms for definition that are used in the implementation and articulation of the total program.

■ *The Conceptual Model*

The original model proposed by Frank Wellman (1962) as a guidance model has been revised several times. The first edition used slightly different terms for the domains (educational, vocational, personal/social) and the levels of learning (called perceptualization, conceptualization, and generalization). In the most recent revision, personal/social is split into two parts. *Social* is defined to include communication, conflict resolution, ethnic/cultural sensitivity, etc. *Personal* becomes a new domain of individual growth (competencies in recreating self through family time, leisure time, recreation, physical wellness, exercise, nutrition). The new model illustrates how the four goals categories, or goals (education, career, social, personal), which represent the domains of content, interact with levels of learning, now called *competencies* (knowledge, skills, attitudes). The third dimension of the model indicates the specific populations to be served. Figure 5.1 shows the conceptual model, to be used as a framework in developing a comprehensive and unique program.

A model, which can also be called a paradigm or a framework, includes specific areas of student results and may exclude others. This model, for example, does not address which agents should be involved in the delivery. It uses the parameters of an educational system to define a way in which all student support professionals can work collaboratively to meet the same or similar goals. In the case of a student support team, a number of different disciplines may be operating under the same conceptual framework. Each member of the student support team should have specific results to offer:

- The school counselor assumes responsibility for the success of each student, using the help of the rest of the team members as needed.
- The school nurse contributes a part of the personal wellness program.
- The social worker ensures that students gain competencies in addressing barriers to learning within the home and community.
- The psychologists work to ensure that all students gain competencies in classroom learning processes and personal problem solving

In addition, informal members of the team, such as community personnel (e.g., recreation specialists and police) are responsible for areas where they are able to contribute to student success. Not all groups within the student support team provide equal attention to each domain, but collectively all domains (education, career, social, and personal) are addressed. Counselors, as advocates, are ultimately responsible for ensuring that each student receives and benefits from the student support program.

The terms *theory, conceptual model,* and *paradigm* are somewhat interchangeable. Each provides parameters, encourages discussions, and provokes research. Each also

- Implies a way of thinking and a way of seeing.
- Is seen as a means of encouraging discourse.
- Has strengths but also limitations (validates some areas, ignores others).
- Offers ways of seeing as well as creating ways of not seeing.
- Provides structure for inclusion and for exclusion.
- Provides a structure for implementation.

■ *Building the Glossary*

The *glossary* is a set of defined terms that provides clear definitions for words and phrases used in the program document. The glossary provides a vehicle for communication among all stakeholders to ensure the program elements are understood; to clarify what is being said; and to identify how, when and where each element applies to the results-based student support program.

In developing the glossary, it is important to consider using definitions provided by known theorists, published conceptual thinkers, or the model builders of our profession. Using accepted definitions not only saves time but also offers opportunities to acquire curriculum already developed, implemented, and evaluated as well as to use research data on the effectiveness of certain strategies. For example, in most student support programs, one set of student competencies to be learned and demonstrated relates to self-esteem. Published model builders in the area of self-esteem include

Robert Reasoner, Jack Canfield, Michele Barbo, and many others. Using a definition of self-esteem from a recognized author aligns the glossary with the published materials used to teach the competencies.

Another area of competency is one in which all students acquire and demonstrate knowledge, skills, and attitudes in learning, including studying and application of what is learned to specific situations. Some of the known theorists and conceptual model builders in this area are Lynda Beemer and Winona Dunne (Study Smarter Not Harder), AVID (SQ3R + the Cornell Notetaking System), Bernice McCarthy (4Mat System), David Kolb (Learning Style Inventory), and Rita and Ken Dunn (Center for Learning Styles, St. John's University, Jamaica, NY).

As the program is developed, other areas with accepted models available include planning, decision making, problem solving, interpersonal relationships, conflict resolution, self-assessment in career interests, aptitudes, values, and wellness. Counseling—both individual and group—and guidance theories, models, and paradigms should also be discussed and defined for the stakeholders in the program. Educators and counselors have developed a unique terminology that may not be clearly understood by many of our constituents. Simple definitions facilitate mutual understanding and collaboration.

■ **ACTIVITY SET 5.1**

Building a Glossary

A. Terms and Phrases	B. Definition Sources
In this column, write a master list of all the words and phrases that you listed in Activities 3.1 and 4.2.	In this column, identify any experts, authors, and/or models you might use as the source of a definition of the word or phrase in column A.

■ REFLECTION

Reflect on your experiences in reviewing the conceptual model of student support programs.

_____

_____

■ SUMMARY

In this chapter we discussed the general definition of conceptual models and the evolution of the Wellman Guidance Model. Terms for definition were compiled from the activities in this and previous chapters. The purpose of the activities in this and the two previous chapters has been to prepare you to explore those areas for which the results-based student support program is held accountable. Areas of accountability are clearly delineated and identification of the program goals is covered in the next chapter.

CHAPTER SIX

Delineating Goals, Standards, and Competencies

Upon completion of this chapter and its activities, you should be able to demonstrate the following competencies:

- **Define and describe the elements of a goal, including the connections with school, district, and state goals**

- **Demonstrate skill in delineating appropriate student competencies from each goal**

- **Demonstrate skill in developing results-based goals that show direct correlations with the statement of mission and philosophy**

- **Compare and describe the differences between goals and standards**

■ *Introduction*

Goals, standards, and competencies are important elements of a results-based program because they define how the program prepares students for future success. Program members must define the specific knowledge, attitudes, and skills that comprise the areas of accountability for the student support program.

Goals and Standards

Goals and standards are statements of intention. They are developed to describe what is to be learned and demonstrated by students graduating from a school or from a program. They specify the desired results or products of the team's efforts. Goals and standards are the program's targets. They validate using resources and staff energies to achieve specific results.

Standards have been developed by the professional organization (ASCA) to define a minimal acceptable level of achievement that professionals in the field of school counseling can agree upon. The current standards are the professional association's first attempt to establish standards for the field of school counseling. They are meant to provide a yardstick for measuring school counseling programs to ensure that all programs nationwide are working from the same set of standards for success.

Goals are unique to each program and are established by the school-based student support staff. Goals may be more extensive than the ASCA standards because they include competencies contributed by the professionals from allied disciplines who are part of a student support team. For example, if nurses are part of the student support team, then it is likely that program goals will include competencies related to good health practices, leading a balanced life, benefits of exercise and good nutrition, and other health-related areas.

Linkages

Program goals *must* be directly aligned with the goals of the school or organization—that is, they must show a relationship with the school's goals. The school's goals must show a relationship with the district's goals, which in turn must show a relationship with the state department of education's goals. The student support program reports data on goal attainment to the school and district administration and also to staff, parents, and students, making both the program and its progress toward goals visible to all stakeholders.

Content

Program goals are expressed in terms of what the students are expected to learn. Therefore, guidance curriculum (content) must be developed to align with the mission, goals, and competencies. The processes used by counselors and other student support professionals to deliver the program are constantly changing in response to the data gathered and are reported within a results framework. No reference is made to the percentage or number of students participating in program activities, only to the number of students who acquire and demonstrate the identified knowledge, attitudes, and skills. The intention is that *each student will acquire the predetermined knowledge, skills, and attitudes.*

Competencies

Competencies are the age- or grade-specific knowledge, skills, and attitudes acquired by students. They are used as indicators to ensure that students are moving toward final goal and mission attainment. These formative data are also used to make sure that what is planned is being achieved. In other words, is the program producing the desired results, and if not, why not? Based on a review of the data, student support staff can and should change their processes to address any deficiencies. In some situations when something is not working, there is a tendency to do it more. However, experience has proven the old adage: "If it isn't working, change it."

Several samples of competencies are listed by goal in Appendix B. They have been amassed from numerous sources, and each has been tested for content and construct validity as well as for developmental appropriateness. Class participants or readers are encouraged to adopt any of the identified competencies in developing a student support program or to create your own. Competencies for each goal do not need to be extensive or cover every possible competency within a goal area; simply select a representative sample of competencies that are indicative of the goals established for the program. When a comprehensive program is implemented, students attain many unplanned competencies as a result of the activities. It is not necessary to list or to measure every competency.

ACTIVITY SET 6.1

Developing Goals

In this activity set, as a class or in small groups, discuss the components of the goals in five examples. In Part A under each example, determine if the components of the education goal meet the criteria listed. In Part B, indicate whether the stated goal satisfies the related ASCA National Standards listed under each example. (Note that the ASCA National Standards combine personal and social into one standard.) In Part C, the group will write goals for an actual or imaginary district or school.

Example 1

Educational Goal

All students in Utopia public schools/PDQ Senior High School will acquire and demonstrate competencies in developing a high school and postsecondary educational program that fulfills their individual learning styles, goals, and objectives that contribute to lifelong learning skills to constructively deal with and contribute to society.

Each student will acquire and demonstrate competencies in

1. Studying and test taking.
2. Utilizing resources, exercising rights and responsibilities, and following rules and regulations.
3. Problem solving and planning educational programs.

Related National Standards

Standard I: Students will acquire the attitudes, knowledge, and skills (competencies) that contribute to effective learning in school and across the life span.

Standard II: Students will complete school with the academic preparation essential to choose from a wide range of substantial postsecondary options, including college.

Standard III: Students will understand the relationship of academic study to the world of work and to life at home and in the community.

A. Evaluate this example based on the following criteria:

1. The goal identifies the clients or population to be addressed.

   _____

   _____

2. The goal is expressed in terms of what students are expected to achieve by the time they are ready to leave the program.

   _____

   _____

3. The goal (or standard) does not define the processes to be used to achieve the goal.

   _____

   _____

4. The goal shows linkage with the mission statement of the school and district.

   _____

   _____

5. Following the goal statement, there is a further definition of specific areas or competency areas encompassed by the goal statement.

   _____

   _____

B. Compare and contrast this example with the related ASCA National Standards.

   _____

   _____

_____

_____

_____

Example 2

Education Goal

The goal for guidance professionals is to assist (help, facilitate, motivate, enable) all students to achieve to their highest potential in the areas of education and lifelong learning.

A. Evaluate this example based on the following criteria:

1. The goal identifies the clients or population to be addressed.

_____

_____

2. The goal is expressed in terms of what students are expected to achieve by the time they are ready to leave the program.

_____

_____

3. The goal (or standard) does not define the processes to be used to achieve the goal.

_____

_____

4. The goal shows linkage with the mission statement of the school and district.

_____

_____

5. Following the goal statement, there is a further definition of specific areas or competency areas encompassed by the goal statement.

_____

_____

B. Compare and contrast this example with the related ASCA National Standards.

_____

_____

_____

_____

_____

_____

Example 3

Career Goal or Standard

All students in Utopia public schools/PDQ Senior High School will acquire and demonstrate competencies in planning and preparing for a career that relates to their career goals and objectives and to their assessed aptitudes, interests, and attitudes/values.

Each student will acquire and demonstrate competencies in

1. Knowledge of self characteristics.

2. Knowledge of the world of work.

3. Career decision making and planning.

4. Finding, keeping and leaving employment.

Related National Standards

Standard I: Students will require the skills to investigate the world of work in relation to knowledge of self and to make informed career decisions.

Standard II: Students will employ strategies to achieve future career goals with success and satisfaction.

Standard III: Students will understand the relationship between personal qualities, education, training, and the world of work.

A. Evaluate this example based on the following criteria:

1. The goal identifies the clients or population to be addressed.

_____

_____

2. The goal is expressed in terms of what students are expected to achieve by the time they are ready to leave the program.

_____

_____

3. The goal (or standard) does not define the processes to be used to achieve the goal.

_____

_____

4. The goal shows linkage with the mission statement of the school and district.

_____

_____

5. Following the goal statement, there is a further definition of specific areas or competency areas encompassed by the goal statement.

_____

_____

B. Describe the ways in which this example does and/or does not satisfy the related ASCA National Standards.

_____

_____

_____

_____

_____

Example 4

Social Goal or Standard

All students in Utopia public schools will acquire and demonstrate competencies in human relationship skills that enhance participation in all life roles, including those of student, worker, family member, and community member. Each student will acquire and demonstrate competencies in

1. Effective interpersonal communication.

2. Utilizing own and others' contributions.

3. Resolving conflict in an appropriate ways.

Related National Standards: Personal/Social

Standard I: Students will acquire the knowledge, attitudes, and interpersonal skills (competencies) to help them understand and respect self and others.

Standard II: Students will make decisions, set goals, and take necessary action to achieve goals.

Standard III: Students will understand safety and survival skills.

A. Evaluate this example based on the following criteria:

1. The goal identifies the clients or population to be addressed.

_____

_____

2. The goal is expressed in terms of what students are expected to achieve by the time they are ready to leave the program.

_____

_____

3. The goal (or standard) does not define the processes to be used to achieve the goal.

_____

_____

4. The goal shows linkage with the mission statement of the school and district.

_____

_____

5. Following the goal statement, there is a further definition of specific areas or competency areas encompassed by the goal statement.

_____

_____

B. Describe the ways in which this example does and/or does not satisfy the related ASCA National Standards.

_____

_____

_____

_____

_____

Example 5

Personal Goal

All students in Utopia public schools will acquire and demonstrate competencies in maintaining a life balanced in learning, family involvement, appropriate nutrition, regular exercise, and community contributions. Each student will acquire and demonstrate the following competencies:

1. Knowledge/awareness of leisure opportunities
2. Knowledge and skills in contributing to the family and to community agendas
3. Planning, implementing, and evaluating an appropriate exercise program
4. Skills in handling personal stress

There are no national standards in the area of personal development.

A. Evaluate this example based on the following criteria:

1. The goal identifies the clients or population to be addressed.

_____

_____

2. The goal is expressed in terms of what students are expected to achieve by the time they are ready to leave the program.

_____

_____

3. The goal (or standard) does not define the processes to be used to achieve the goal.

_____

_____

4. The goal shows linkage with the mission statement of the school and district.

_____

_____

5. Following the goal statement, there is a further definition of specific areas or competency areas encompassed by the goal statement.

_____

_____

B. Describe the ways in which this example does and/or does not satisfy the related ASCA National Standards.

_____

_____

_____

C. Writing Goals

Either individually or in a small group, develop program goals for an identified actual or imagined district and/or school by using the previous examples as guides or by creating new ones that best fit the school's or district's learning community. Individuals are encouraged to work at this task in the way that is best for the class structure: (1) work with others on selecting and developing competencies for each goal, or (2) divide the group or class and have one or more individuals work on different goals and then come together to describe their efforts.

1. Educational Goal

_____

_____

_____

_____

_____

_____

_____

_____

2. Career Goal

_____

_____

_____

_____

_____

_____

_____

_____

_____

3. Social Goal

_____

_____

_____

_____

_____

_____

_____

_____

4. Personal Goal

_____

_____

_____

_____

_____

_____

_____

_____

_____

■ REFLECTION

Use this space to reflect on what you have learned and what you think of the exercises in which you participated.

_____

_____

_____

_____

_____

_____

■ SUMMARY

In this chapter the definition and criteria of goals were presented as was the importance of ensuring the relationships of school and district goals with the student-support program goals. In addition, student participants developed their own goals in four areas or domains: education, career development, social skills, and personal development. Each goal was then defined through delineated sets of competencies that give more direct directions for results. The next chapter addresses how the program will be managed, including decisions on program and individual accountability.

PART THREE

Implementation

CHAPTER SEVEN

Management Systems

Upon completion of this chapter and its activities, you should be able to demonstrate the following competencies:

- **Know the differences between management for results and management of processes and/or services**

- **Identify the ways individuals might be assigned and indicate the positive and limited consequences of each method**

- **Use consensus building to arrive at agreements**

▪ *Introduction*

Many student support programs are managed through assignment of activities listed in a role-and-function document or in a job description adopted by the district. Use of role-and-function documents and job descriptions for employing personnel assumes that all professionals with the same title, such as school counselor or psychologist, are equally competent in the same skills. Thus, counselors and other student support professionals from the first day of work must conform to the expectations of a system designed in a traditional format. Many of the items listed in a role-and-function document have little to do with student results; they are primarily responses to system needs. For this situation to change, the counselors and other student support staff must specify their own contributions and accept responsibility for producing student results. One way this can happen is to reorient the management system from services to student results.

■ *Management of the Results-Based Student Support Program*

Managing a results-based student support program calls for a different set of managerial skills than those used in a traditional system (Kiersey & Bates, 1972). It is the opposite of managing the role and function of staff members or of services. The administrator in charge is primarily concerned with student results, not with the processes used to achieve the results. The manager leaves these "how-to" decisions to those who are accountable for the results. Many conceptualizers of management systems—Douglas McGregor, Rensis Likert, and Warren Bennis—make the case that a system dedicated to results must allow the producers of the results to decide the best means to achieve them. This process of individual accountability for processes allows individual strengths to be used, thus recognizing professional skill differences.

For a results-based program, the management functions identified by Kiersey and Bates (1972) offer an appropriate manager-producer set of functions for both program and individual accountability. These functions allow student support staff members to identify the varied contributions of each member of the team in attaining student results. Well-defined individual responsibilities (accountability) are the hallmark of the student support program. Staff will begin to notice the need for collaboration to enfranchise partners in the student support efforts. This broadening of the student support team then allows for more expansive and effective student support curricula. An example of this preplanned management of duties follows.

Student Support Team	Manager/Administrator/Director
(Counselor, psychologist, social worker, nurse and other specialists)	
1. Produces and presents results agreements; arrives at consensus with the person in charge.	1. Reviews results agreements, negotiates, and arrives at consensus
2. Produces and presents plans to achieve results; reaches consensus.	2. Audits and accepts plans to achieve results; reaches consensus.
3. Implements plans and produces progress reports as scheduled.	3. Monitors activities and notes progress.
4. Produces assessable evidence of results attained, reflects on data, and develops plans to use data for improvement.	4. Audits evidence of results, reviews reflection, provides input, and validates progress.
5. Acquires new competencies and updates skills.	5. Coaches to encourage new competencies; provides opportunities for advanced training.

The unspoken factor in management responsibility is the need for mutual appreciation between manager and student support team. They must work together, agree on the focus and desired outcomes of the program, and forge a working relationship that allows flexibility and change in dealing with processes that are not working.

Organization and Assignments

To implement the management system, decisions regarding the organization and assignment of counselors should be made prior to the next step in program implementation, the development of results agreements. These decisions allow the student support team to maintain the current structure or to restructure to provide a better match between resources and planned-for results. In traditional school counseling programs, counselors are assigned a caseload of students for record keeping, monitoring student progress toward promotion or graduation, and ensuring that each student has an assigned adult, to discuss educational and personal concerns. When the student support team begins to address the range of results and the whole student population, the traditional management system becomes cumbersome, inefficient, and ripe for change.

Time spent in planning by the entire team provides the vehicle needed to design and implement a program that will meet the individual goals of each student. Planning allows the student support team to better define individual contributions and responsibilities and helps produce a better fit between expectations and meeting the needs of all students in the areas of learning to learn, learning to work, learning to relate to others, and learning to develop and maintain personal wellness. In a results-based program, responsibility for specific results and/or specific areas does not necessarily mean the manager will automatically be performing all the activities personally; other members of the student support team, faculty, community members, or others may actually work with the students to accomplish the results. The manager is responsible for ensuring that the results have been accomplished. This management approach to guidance requires teamwork because others are often providing the competencies for which the manager is responsible. The manager collects and reports the results for accountability purposes.

If a school has only one counselor (the current norm at many elementary schools), then by necessity this counselor is responsible for all the students. In such cases it becomes even more important to include others in a student support team in order to reach each student. Currently there is no available research that supports any specific counselor-student ratio or assignment. However, when a school has two or more counselors, there are a number of different ways to structure student support personnel assignments:

- *Counselors are assigned students alphabetically.* This system, which equalizes caseloads, divides the number of students by the number of counselors, then divides the alphabet to match an equal number of students for each counselor so that the counselor has students from each grade level. Counselors must obtain essential information for all grade levels, including all school requirements as well as college and university requirements and community resources.

- *Counselors stay with the same class through all the grades.* In this system, counselors are responsible for the same students throughout their schooling until they graduate. Counselors must stay current with requirements for only one grade at a time, learning or renewing knowledge necessary for that grade level. For example, counselors working with senior students who have not had seniors for four years may need updating on the university requirements, post–high school opportunities, and senior activities that may have changed dramatically in the interim.

- *Counselors have a permanent grade level assignment.* Counselors only deal with one grade level at a time, becoming in effect an expert for that grade. They gain deep knowledge of the grade-specific courses, expectations, teachers, and developmental tasks.

- *Counselors are assigned by teacher.* Each counselor is responsible for assisting the students in each of a teacher's classes to attain specific results, such as learning how to learn; establishing, implementing, and evaluating personal goals; and learning how to prepare résumés and college applications. Competencies are "assigned" to certain classes or curriculum areas, and the counselor works with teachers to ensure that each student attains them.

- *Counselors are assigned to families.* A counselor is assigned to a family when the first child in the family enrolls in school and adds each sibling as he/she enrolls. The families become the caseload.

- *Counselors have no assigned caseload.* Counselors work with any or all students on specific needs. Students can select the counselor they wish to consult on an as-needed basis.

- *Counselors are assigned by goal area.* The counselor is accountable for one or more of the goal areas (depending upon the number of counselors available). One might assume responsibility for the educational goal, one for the career goal, one for the interpersonal goal, and one for the personal development goal. (It is important to note that being accountable means managing and not necessarily doing. In managing, you develop a plan and call on colleagues and others to help. You might use parents, peer tutors, teachers, and others in implementing your plans.)

- *Counselors have a combination of assignments.* Combinations include a caseload plus a goal; a smaller caseload plus handling all potential dropouts; a caseload that includes only special needs students or other designated groups. This assignment pattern sometimes evolves in response to funding limits for specific categories such as drug counselor, vocational position, school safety, Title I, and the like.

- *Counselors in the upper grades are assigned by student majors,* such as college, military, technical, and so on. Counselors can concentrate on specific aspects of post–high school planning, seeking options, resources, and experiences that apply to identified students. For example, the counselor might secure part-time work as a candy striper for a student interested in medical or hospital-related careers.

- *Counselors are assigned by teacher advisor or homeroom.* Some schools assign a teacher to act as a contact person, advisor, or mentor to students and meet with them on a regular basis. The counselor works directly with these teachers and assumes responsibility for their assigned students.

When a school has more than two counselors, the unique strengths of each member must be considered in planning for specific results. A team member who can work in an area of choice will be motivated; using that person's strengths leads to more energy and a sense of belonging. However, it is important to cover each element or piece of the program to ensure that students will acquire all competencies specified in the results-based program. Portions of the assignment that are not chosen will necessarily be shared.

A "counselor-of-the-day" strategy can help break away from traditional time constraints. This strategy assigns one counselor each day to address crisis situations, accept student referrals, enroll new students, take phone calls, and handle routine tasks. This allows other counselors time to create and pilot new processes for achieving student results. Remember, there is no right way to assign areas of accountability to team members. *The way you choose for your situation is the right way for you.* However, it is important to know why you choose a specific configuration so that if things don't work out the way they are intended to, there is a "fault-tree" to retrace the steps taken, assess the problem, and make new decisions.

■ **ACTIVITY SET 7.1**

Assigning Students and Tasks

A. Identify the advantages and disadvantages (for students) of these methods of assigning students before selecting one or more for your program.

1. Counselors are assigned students alphabetically.

Advantages	Disadvantages

2. Counselors stay with the same class through all the grades.

Advantages	Disadvantages

3. Counselors have a permanent grade level assignment.

Advantages	Disadvantages

4. Counselors are assigned by teacher.

Advantages	Disadvantages

5. Counselors are assigned to families.

Advantages	Disadvantages

6. Counselors have no assigned caseload.

Advantages	Disadvantages

7. Counselors are assigned by goal area.

Advantages	Disadvantages

8. Counselors have a combination of assignments.

Advantages	Disadvantages

9. Counselors in the upper grades are assigned by student majors.

Advantages	Disadvantages

10. Counselors are assigned by teacher advisor or homeroom teacher.

Advantages	Disadvantages

B. From the preceding list, make a selection for your (actual or imagined) school and in the space below provide a rationale for the choices made:

Choice for assignment:

Rationale (pros and cons):

_____

_____

_____

_____

_____

C. Discuss in class or in small groups the different ways in which other student support professionals might be assigned to best utilize their expertise with students. Include school psychologist, school social worker, nurse, health aide, and other specialists you would include on a student support team. For discussion purposes, assume that you are not constrained by funding, legislative requirements (excluding special education laws), or other external factors.

D. List the tasks/duties that should be assigned in writing to each professional on the student support team. *Do not include assumed tasks or volunteer duties.* Assumed tasks are those tasks that counselors and other student support team members have always done because they assumed it was their duty. Because they are not put down in writing, they are considered assumed (optional). In a results-based program, the only assigned tasks or duties are ones the administrator puts in writing, all others are considered assumed or self-determined.

_____

_____

_____

_____

_____

_____

_____

_____

_____

_____

_____

_____

_____

_____

_____

_____

Now go back to the list of duties and check to see if any of the tasks you have entered are assumed and not assigned in writing. Assigned tasks might be answering telephones, bus or lunch duty, or filling in for a teacher who becomes ill or has been assigned to attend an off-campus location. Cross out any assumed tasks. You should have only assigned tasks left on your list. Write after each assigned task the professional on the team who should do it, making an effort to ensure that the total time expended on assigned tasks is relatively equal. Remember, all assumed responsibilities should relate directly to student results. Assigned tasks are process-determined by someone else, are related to a school system need.

E. This activity will determine how the different areas of the student support program curriculum will be assigned to ensure that each student will acquire the competencies.

1. Class members form one or more teams, and each team chooses a facilitator to conduct the meeting activity.

2. In a "go around" each person is asked to describe her or his strengths, and other group members give feedback on their perception of the person's strengths.

3. When each person, including the chair, has had a turn, group members request their first and second choice for managing a specific domain of results. Remember, this means planning and managing the activities, not necessarily doing all the work. It should be a team approach. Each manager assumes accountability for results in the domain selected; all are expected to contribute toward achieving the results. The domain of results, not the people, are being managed.

F. Now decide who should be the manager for each results area. In each case, write a brief rationale for your decision.

1. Educational domain

   Who? _____

   Rationale _____

2. Career domain

   Who? _____

   Rationale _____

3. Social domain

   Who? _____

   Rationale _____

4. Personal domain

   Who? _____

   Rationale _____

G. Other results areas—such as health needs, handicapping conditions, career center/ROP, Career-to-Work, Special Education—may be needed for specific students/programs to fulfill special funding requirements. Identify these special requirements and give a rationale for each decision.

Specific Area _____

Rationale _____

_____

Specific Area _____

Rationale _____

_____

Specific Area _____

Rationale _____

_____

■ REFLECTION

Please take time to reflect on the work you have done in this chapter on assigning students and tasks to the counselors and other professionals on the student support team.

_____

_____

_____

_____

_____

_____

_____

_____

_____

■ SUMMARY

This chapter was a first look at how the management of the results-based student support program is conducted. Program expectations were presented, and was presented different methods of matching professional expertise with expectations. An activity demonstrated how individuals choose their areas of contribution; then you listed all assigned tasks identified in writing from the administration. The next chapter will focus on developing an accountability agreement for delivering specific student results.

CHAPTER EIGHT

Results Agreements

Upon completion of this chapter and its activities, you should be able to demonstrate the following competencies:

- **Understand the advantages of having all the professionals on the student support team develop their own results agreement**
- **Skills in developing a results agreement**
- **Skills in negotiating the agreement with the administration in charge**

Introduction

The *results agreement* contains the individual counselor's job description. Results agreements delineate the specific responsibilities and contributions of each student support team member. Each individual's agreement is shared with all student support team members and negotiated to ensure that all aspects of the program are being addressed. After the team agreements are reached, each counselor's agreement is reviewed and negotiated with the administrator in charge. The results agreement consists of a set of results to be delivered by the counselor (or student support professional) for students, parents, and teaching staff and a set of tasks assigned by the administration. It is a statement of the individual professional's accountability for student, parent, and staff results.

Advantages of Results Agreements

There are several reasons and advantages for using a results agreement:

- Each student support team member has the opportunity to determine her or his own job description (formerly known as the role and function).
- Results are negotiated separately from the activities used for delivery, thereby allowing flexibility in activities while keeping the results constant.

- Planned-for student results are presented to the administration, staff, parents, and students as priorities of the guidance program.

- The results agreement declares the areas of accountability for each student support program professionals.

- The agreement is written to identify the competencies that each student will attain through the efforts of the student support program and illustrates the link between the mission and goals of the program, the school, and the district.

- It sets the stage for accountability and visibility of the results the student support team achieves. (Note that the agreement is addressed not only to the local school administration but also to the district office).

- The administrator monitors the contributions of the student support team as they relate to the school's goals and thus confirms the importance of the program within the functioning of the entire school. The program is no longer marginalized but becomes an integral part of each student's total educational program.

Results agreements focus the administration's expectations for the counselor/student support staff by pointing out the potential impact the student support program can have when it is planned and managed by student support professionals. The agreements are stated in terms of results, not activities, so activities can be planned, adapted, or changed whenever the expected results are not being achieved. The agreements emphasize accountability for student results, not simply for the completion of activities. This self-generated responsibility increases the credibility and the status of the counselor as a skilled professional.

Further, the results agreements help the student support team address the specifics of collaboration by recognizing the responsibilities and interdependency of each participant in the results agreement negotiation. When activities are approached with a vague goal of involving others but are without specific targeted outcomes or descriptions of each participant's responsibilities, effectiveness is limited. The articulation of outcomes among all student support team members both clarifies expectations and engenders the support of the administration toward cooperation and collaboration among participants. It is more likely that all contributors will be supported and will carry through with the agreement if the administration is fully informed and signs off on it beforehand.

Another distinct advantage of the results agreement is it gives individual professionals the freedom to identify specific outcomes and expectations for themselves. The section of the results agreement focusing on self-development invites professionals to identify knowledge and skill areas they wish to gain or improve. The support for further training, materials, or other resources is built in as a logical part of the continuing evaluation and improvement of the program's contributions. It is not unusual to request funding, time off, or other administrative support and be granted the time and resources to participate in growth opportunities when there is a connection between skills to be gained and the desired student competencies.

The results agreement may help to define the student outcomes of activities that are already occurring in a program, but most will find that the results agreement is helpful in planning more expansive duties to address domains of responsibility that have been under addressed. Results agreements will also focus the student support staff on more systematic planning of curriculum in order to achieve better results.

■ *Content of the Results Agreement*

In developing results agreements, think in terms of expected outcomes for each discipline represented on the student support team and how team members might choose to achieve their own stated outcomes. This will help later to guide the student support team toward effective and comprehensive activities that weave participants together in a coordinated team approach. For example, if a counselor plans to teach how to make healthy, balanced lifestyle decisions, then coordinating the results agreement with similar intentions expressed by the school nurse makes sense. Subsequently, the counselor and nurse may choose to work together to jointly meet their agreed-upon student outcomes. In some cases, such as with school psychologists and social workers, primary results may fall within the "referred student" section of the results agreement because they assume responsibility for students referred to them because of difficulties in learning within the classroom or outside distracters that interfere with learning.

The results agreement consists of several sections, each an integral part of a comprehensive program:

1. *Program results* The first and most important part of any results agreement is the Program Results section. Here the counselor identifies the specific outcomes for all students—or all assigned students or specific groups of students. A comprehensive program ensures that all students will benefit from the program, so it is important that all students are addressed in the results agreement of one or more counselors or other student support staff members. Several examples of program results statements follow:

- All ninth grade students shall acquire and demonstrate knowledge of the high school graduation requirements and skills in planning a program of studies that leads to graduation.

- All seventh grade students will demonstrate skills in using standard note taking skills for completing assignments and test preparation.

- All fourth grade students will describe and demonstrate skills in setting goals in the personal and social domain.

- All students in special education classes will demonstrate basic organizational skills needed for learning. (Refer to sample results agreements in Activity Set 8.1 for additional examples.)

2. *Referred students results* This set of results addresses students who are referred to the counselor/psychology/nurse by themselves or others for personal or school concerns. These concerns may include not getting along in the classroom or playground and study behavior that suggests assistance is required (attention or time-on-task deficits), or the referral may be generated by a parent who requests help with out-of-classroom distracters that interfere with the student's success. The following is an example of a results statement in this category:

Each student referred for personal concerns by self or others (e.g., teacher, parent, friend) will identify the problem, appropriate alternatives to address the problem, complete a plan to remedy the problem, implement the plan, evaluate the results, and return to discuss the results and next steps with the student support team member.

3. *Staff results* All student support personnel are committed to supporting both students and classroom teachers to increase academic achievement. Student support staff members provide a source of assistance for teachers in facilitating the learning process by offering mentoring and in-service activities, facilitating teacher/parent meetings, and consistently working to improve the learning climate within the classroom and the school. Student support staff frequently act as a sounding board for teachers exploring new ideas for teaching and learning or seeking strategies to help specific students learn. It is also important that teachers become active participants in the guidance program, providing information, referrals, support, curriculum alignment, and other contributions to support student learning. Finding ways to collaborate with teachers and other staff members is a valuable addition to the guidance program.

4. *Parent results* Most student support administrators agree that the counselor has the responsibility for planning, implementing, and evaluating programs for parent participation in activities connected with student academic achievement, including parent education–related programs, such as learning how to help your child study, identifying home learning styles, creating home learning environments, learning about child development indicators, making classroom visits most productive for parent and child, and so on. The inclusion of staff and parent results validates the involvement of all the responsible adults who are invested in helping students succeed. The act of including others in efforts to reach each student makes the desired results more attainable. Research findings are clear on the importance of parent involvement for student success, and parents can be more effective if they are provided with information and tools. It is unconscionable to profess that you want all students to succeed and ignore the most valuable resource for making that happen.

It is the counselor's job to ensure that parents have the opportunity and preparation to actively assist their children in the educational experience. However, when addressing parents and staff, it is essential to remember that *the student is the primary client.* The student support staff is responsible not for meeting parents' mental health needs, but rather for working together with the other caring adults in a student's life to ensure the student's success. This important distinction protects the time and resources of the student support program for the sole benefit of the student and his or her educational success.

5. *Self-development results* Student support staff must maintain a high level of professional aptitude. There is no such thing as a status quo in today's world, and advances in computer science, telecommunications, and biotechnology have the potential to dramatically change the guidance programs of the future. Some current changes include multiple uses of technology to facilitate parent involvement in student education, including scheduling high school classes and teacher selection via phone or computer, parent portals to review grades and communicate with teachers on a weekly or as-needed basis, distance learning for high school students, interactive video conferencing, and virtual high schools. To allow one's professional skills to lapse is to become obsolete.

Self-development is the hallmark of professionalism and includes active participation in professional associations, attendance at annual conferences, and periodic training in new areas. Although additional training often becomes part of a requirement for renewing credentials, it is the counselor's individual responsibility to remain current in the discipline. By listing their main areas of interest for the year, counselors make the administrator aware of training opportunities needed for maintaining an up-to-date guidance program. Areas such as changing university requirements, bully-proofing a school, crisis management, mediation, peer tutoring, and the like have all received attention in the last few years, and every guidance department needs one or more professionals trained in each of these areas. Coordination of requests for professional development among team members facilitates growth by providing an avenue for sharing content from workshops with colleagues, with parents, and with other staff members. The self-development section of the results agreement makes training needs visible and validates counselors' intention to continue their professional development.

6. *Assigned tasks* Assigned tasks are duties specified by the administrator in writing that assist administrators to achieve their results. In fulfilling assigned tasks, the student support professional is responsible only for implementing the process, not for assessing the results attained. The administrator who assigned the task is responsible to assess the results attained since she or he determined the process. It is important to note that all educators share some responsibility for processes that help a school function and/or are necessary for student safety. However, counselors should not be expected to assume more than an equal share of the time or responsibility for these routine tasks.

This last section opens the door for communication and negotiation to ensure that counselors are not assigned an unequal number of tasks unrelated to guidance. For example, an administrator may believe that "testing" is the counselor's job. However, using the results agreement as the point of discussion, counselors can point out that using testing results, communicating with parents and staff about the significance of test results for individual students, and using analysis to help improve test results, planning appropriate program placement for students, and similar tasks are all aspects of testing that fall within the counseling arena. On the other hand, administering tests, recording test results in student records, and other such tasks are basically clerical jobs that logically belong in the office of administration. Counselors have traditionally assumed many clerical tasks in order to help maintain a school program, but when they are analyzed in terms of the student results they provide, these tasks have no place in the counseling program. Requiring that such responsibilities be recorded in writing at the beginning of the school year makes it easier for counselors to plan their schedules, and it becomes obvious to counselors and administrators alike when counselors are regularly doing more than their fair share.

■ **ACTIVITY SET 8.1**

Developing a Results Agreement

Please sit together in small groups to do this activity. When members of a team work together in forming the elements of a program, it facilitates future networking and sharing progress reports.

A. Please review the following examples of results agreements. Discuss the wording that identifies projected student, staff, and parent results or identifies competencies that students, parents, staff or self will acquire. In the next part of the activity, each member of the group will develop a tentative agreement for a selected learning community.

Sample 1

HIGH SCHOOL RESULTS AGREEMENT

To: _____, Administrator　　Date: _____

_____　　School

From: _____, Counselor　　Date: _____

RE: Results Agreement for ___to___ school year

cc: _____, Area Superintendent

cc: _____, Coordinator of Student Support Programs

I will make the following contributions to the students, parents, and staff during the _____ to _____school year.

1.0 Program Results:

> 1.1 Each student in grades 9–12 will identify graduation requirements and will describe which requirements he/she has fulfilled or has yet to meet.

> 1.2 Each student in grades 9–12 will demonstrate skills in utilizing college and financial aid software to complete a career and post–high school educational plan.

> 1.3 Each student in grades 9–12 will demonstrate skills
> in completing and updating a résumé;
> in completing job and college/university applications;
> in using personal competence to provide a service for the community;
> in group membership.

2.0 Referred Students Results: Each student referred for individual or group counseling by self or another shall
- Identify the problem characteristics.
- List alternative solutions and consequences of each.
- Choose a solution and complete a plan to follow through.
- Follow through on plan.
- Evaluate their results.
- If necessary, will try another solution.

3.0 Parent Results: The parents of all students in grades 9–11 will demonstrate skills in using college and financial aid software to help their child to complete a post–high school career and educational plan.

4.0 Staff Results: All teachers will describe or list student behavior that might reflect abuse.

5.0 Self Results: I will acquire competencies in recognizing and assisting students referred for behaviors that might reflect abuse.

6.0 Assigned Tasks: The administrator must put assigned tasks on the results agreement in writing.

Sample 2

MIDDLE SCHOOL RESULTS AGREEMENT

TO: _____, Administrator   Date:_____

_____   Middle School

From: _____, Counselor   Date:_____

RE: Results Agreement for ___to___ school year

cc: _____, Area Superintendent

cc: _____, Coordinator of Student Support Programs

I will make the following contributions to students, parents, and staff during the _____ to _____ school year.

1.0 Program Results: Students will demonstrate the following competencies:

   1.1 Each eighth grade student shall
   - Describe her/his preferred learning style and matching study skills.
   - List the high school graduation requirements and select a four (4) year course of study leading to graduation.
   - Demonstrate skills in using the computer search software to select a career(s) of choice.
   - Utilize skills in managing personal time to allow for school, study, responsibilities, and leisure.

   1.2 Each seventh grade student shall
   - Demonstrate personal problem-solving skills.
   - Demonstrate skills in organization of time and school materials.
   - Utilize skills in group membership.
   - Demonstrate knowledge of when and how to assist a peer with personal problems or issues.

   1.3 Each sixth grade student shall
   - Demonstrate skills in studying.
   - Utilize skills in using available resources in learning, positive work habits, and relating to others.
   - Utilize personal skills in contributing to school activities.

2.0 Referred Students Results: Each student referred to me by self or others shall describe the problem characteristics, list alternative solutions and the consequences of each, choose a solution, complete a plan to correct the problem, follow the plan, and evaluate the conclusion.

3.0 Parents Results: The parents of all sixth grade students will use the knowledge of their student's preferred learning style in assisting with homework.

4.0 Staff Results: The teachers of all sixth grade students will identify the student's preferred learning style.

5.0 Self Results: I will acquire competencies in selecting and using learning style assessments for sixth graders.

6.0 Assigned Tasks: The following are tasks that have been assigned to me:

   6.1 _____

   _____

   _____

6.2 _____

_____

_____

Sample 3

ELEMENTARY SCHOOL RESULTS AGREEMENT

TO: _____, Administrator   Date: _____

_____   Elementary School

From: _____, Counselor   Date: _____

RE: Results Agreement for _____ to _____ school year

cc: _____, Area Superintendent

cc: _____, Coordinator of Student Support Programs

I am going to make the following contributions to the students, parents, and staff during the _____ school year.

1.0 Program Results: Students will acquire and demonstrate the following competencies:

   1.1 Each fifth grade student shall demonstrate knowledge and skills in
     • Resolving interpersonal conflict.
     • Preparing for and successfully completing standardized and teacher made tests.
     • Studying and completing homework.

   1.2 Each fourth grade student shall demonstrate knowledge and skills in
     • Organizing her/his school materials.
     • Problem solving.
     • Effective group membership.

   1.3 Each third grade student shall demonstrate skills in studying and preparing for and taking standardized tests.

2.0 Referred Students Results: Each student referred for individual or group counseling shall demonstrate the following competencies in personal problem solving:
     • Identify/describe the problem and the characteristics of the problem.
     • Discuss alternative solutions and the consequences of each in solving the problem.
     • Choose a solution and complete a plan to solve the problem, including a timeline and evaluation.

3.0 Parent Results: The parents of all second grade students shall demonstrate knowledge of how to construct a home learning environment and establish rituals to enhance their child's academic achievement.

4.0 Staff Results: Each teacher shall identify skills in managing playground conflict.

5.0 Self Results: I shall renew and acquire new skills in working with parents to help them assist their child in studying.

6.0 Assigned Tasks: I have been assigned the following tasks to complete and duties to maintain:

6.1 Lunch duty
6.2 Membership on the SST
6.3 Filling in for teachers who are ill or called away for emergencies

Sample 4

HIGH SCHOOL RESULTS AGREEMENT
TO: _____, Administrator   Date:_____
_____   High School
From: _____, Counselor   Date:_____
RE: Results Agreement for _____ to _____ school year
cc:_____, Area Superintendent
cc:_____, Coordinator of Student Support Programs

I am going to make the following contributions to students, parents, and staff during the _____school year.

1.0 Program Results:

1.1 Each ninth grade and tenth grade student shall demonstrate study and test-taking skills.

1.2 Each eleventh and twelfth grade student identified as requiring assistance in completing schoolwork shall acquire and apply specific competencies related to improving classroom performance.

1.3 Each student in grades 9–12 shall identify personal academic skills and shall develop a plan to increase academic achievement.

1.4 Each student in grades 9–12 shall demonstrate competencies in applying for college admission and in identifying eligibility and applying for financial aid.

2.0 Referred Students Results: Each student referred for counseling by self or another shall

- Identify the characteristics of the presenting problem.
- List alternative solutions and consequences of each.
- Choose a solution and complete a plan to follow through.

3.0 Assigned Students Results: Each student assigned for monitoring academic progress shall

3.1 Acquire and demonstrate the competencies delineated in the student support program at the appropriate grade level.

3.2 Enroll and successfully complete courses leading to graduation and to a career of choice.

3.3 Have an up-to-date educational and career plan that has been approved by the parent or guardian.

3.4 Demonstrate appropriate progress toward gaining competencies needed to pass the exit exam.

4.0 Parent Results: Parents of all students in grades 9 and 11 shall demonstrate skills in using available career center resources to assist their student in completing a post–high school career and educational plan.

5.0 Staff Results: All teachers shall identify the learning style of each student who is not performing academically up to expectations and identify two teaching strategies that match the identified learning style.

6.0 Self Results: I shall acquire competencies in helping students to learn test-taking skills.

7.0 Assigned Tasks:

7.1 _____

_____

7.2 _____

_____

7.3 _____

_____

7.4 _____

_____

B. Next, using Worksheet 8.1 (Developing a Results Agreement), create a tentative agreement for the contributions you would choose to make as a member of a student support team.

C. After completing a results agreement for your assumed responsibilities, have someone else in your class review it for the following:

1. Are all statements related only to results, with no processes for attaining the results indicated in the statement?

Comments: _____

_____

2. Are all competencies stated in demonstrable terms, such as what students must know (list, describe, identify) or what they can demonstrate (articulate verbally, skill they can produce, something they can write, a skill someone else can observe)?

Comments: _____

_____

3. Do results stated for adults (staff, parents, self) relate to student results, such as improved learning skills, identification of resources, and support from others?

Comments: _____

_____

4. Does the time needed to complete all assigned tasks account for 10% or less of the counselor's work time?

Comments: _____

_____

5. Which assigned tasks could be renegotiated with an administrator to produce more positive results? For example, instead of having lunch duty, could the counselor be "on duty" in the guidance center during lunch so students would have access to a counselor and needed information without having to get dismissed from class during the regular school day?

Comments: _____

_____

■ REFLECTION

Reflect on your experiences in reviewing the use of results agreements to define your contributions.

_____

_____

_____

_____

_____

_____

_____

_____

_____

■ SUMMARY

This chapter presents the concept of using *results agreements* to encourage student support professionals to interact with each other, to determine program responsibilities, and then to write each job description based on the group agreement for division of labor. The results agreement addresses six areas: student program results, referred student results, parent results, staff results, self-development results, and assigned duties and tasks. Once the results agreement is completed, it is reviewed with the administrator and planning begins. Finding unique ways to ensure success for each student in academic achievement and self-development is not a new paradigm, but it is particularly effective when all student support team members are focusing on the same goals. The next chapter addresses needs assessment as a means of auditing the program progress as well as identifying problems to be addressed.

Developing a Results Agreement

TO: _____, Administrator   Date: _____

_____, School

From: _____, Counselor   Date: _____

RE: Results Agreement for _____ school year

cc: _____, Area Superintendent

cc: _____, Coordinator of Student Support Programs

RE: My Results Agreement for _____ (Year)

I am going to make the following contributions to students, parents, and staff during the _____ school year.

1.0 Program Results:

_____

_____

_____

_____

2.0 Referred Students:

_____

_____

_____

3.0 Staff Results:

_____

_____

_____

_____

4.0 Parent Results:

_____

_____

_____

_____

_____

5.0 Self-Development:

_____

_____

_____

_____

6.0 Assigned Duties:

_____

_____

_____

_____

_____

CHAPTER NINE

Needs Assessment Data

Upon completion of this chapter and its activities, you should be able to demonstrate the following competencies:

- **Identify needs data**
- **Know where data sources are located**

■ *Introduction*

Needs are what is required to reach a specific objective, goal, or outcome. Needs are the discrepancy between the current state of being and the desired outcome; they are the difference between what is and what should be. Needs are also the data that drive the processes of change. The wider the gap between the desired condition and the current condition, the greater the need and the greater urgency for intervention with new methods.

Student support professionals consistently identify needs in their daily work life. When they interact with a student, they can isolate needs and address them on a one-to-one basis. If a large number of students are identified with the same needs, the professional may choose to work with groups of students or use other means to close the gap between what is and what is expected.

However, needs assessment of student achievement depends on having a program that clearly defines expected results. *Student results are the focus of the results-based student support program.* The mission, philosophy, goals, and competencies, all of which are directly aligned with school and district needs, are specifically related to student academic achievement.

■ *Sources of Needs Data*

Needs data are found in numerous sources, including the following:

- Grade point averages
- Failures of students in specific courses

- Attendance rates, truancy rates
- Incidents of vandalism
- Teacher and school referrals for discipline
- Parent involvement
- Teacher absences
- Standardized test scores
- Involvement in extra curricular activities
- Community service

and (at the secondary school level):

- ACT/SAT preparation
- Number of students taking tests successfully
- Number of students applying for and going on to higher education

The actual data for identifying program needs required to make changes in the delivery of program content are often available in the school's data pool used to develop the school profile. A major function of the student support team is the collection and use of student needs data related to the delineated program results.

Another source of data is the teacher. Time spent either in communicating with teachers in the teachers' lounge or in classroom observation can clarify the support needs of classroom teachers and of students. Another possible means of data collection is survey instruments, such as a test anxiety survey or problem-solving quiz, which can be used within a classroom and can generate data that can be used to design appropriate classroom curricula. Teachers willingly provide observational data on deficits in educational skills that are evident in students' classwork and become advocates of the program when counselors respond to their input.

■ *Student Needs Versus Student Wants*

It is very important that the difference between *student needs* and *student wants* is clearly recognized. The following are some examples of student wants assessments:

1. A survey asks students how much help they need in a variety of areas, such as making friends, studying, getting along at home, paying attention in class, and the like. Unless these areas are specific to your predetermined outcomes, they are "wants."

2. A survey asks for student input on the school and/or the student support program. Questions such as "What help would you like to have from the guidance counselors?" or "Which of the following would you like for your school: longer lunch periods, time to study, choosing your own teachers, more voice in the student government, or having one day a school month off to go on a field trip?" are not relevant for program directions.

3. Similarly, there are numerous surveys available for students to assess their attitudes about many aspects of the learning experiences. These usually ask, "How do you feel about . . . ?" or "How useful to you is . . . ?" Unless the attitudes being assessed are stated in the student

competencies section of your student support plan, the data collected are irrelevant. In other words, there is no significant reason to collect data that will not be of use in meeting specified student results.

On the other hand, needs assessments that measure a gap in results allow the student support team to coordinate a program approach to meeting needs. A sample high school needs assessment is provided in Appendix D (The Individual Guidance Assessment). Feel free to utilize all or part of this instrument to help in your planning. When you use needs assessment instruments, check whether you are asking for student wants or identifying gaps in results. You are also encouraged to go to the section on student monitoring in Chapter 11 for more examples of needs data sources.

■ ACTIVITY SET 9.1

Connecting Needs Assessment to Program Results

The purpose of this group of activities is to connect the needs assessment process to program results as well as to both team and individual accountability. These activities are best done in small groups.

A. Refer to the Results Agreement you wrote in Chapter 8 and identify a specific result you would like to work on. It can be any one that you are willing to share with your group. Now write in the proposed result. (Example: Students will know how to study.)

_____

_____

_____

B. Next, identify where and how you might get results information at your work site. (Example: Ask teachers to identify students who are failing, survey parents, review student records.)

_____

_____

_____

_____

C. List the kinds of data you can use to establish needs. (Examples: A list of students who are getting Ds and Fs; teachers identify students not doing their homework.)

_____

_____

_____

_____

_____

D. Now take turns sharing what you have identified with other group members. Add or delete ideas to what you have contributed.

■ REFLECTION

Comment on your reactions, progress, and thoughts about the process thus far and about how your group is working together.

_____

_____

_____

_____

_____

■ SUMMARY

This chapter examines the paradigm of needs assessment. Needs are the data gaps between what is and what should be. Put another way, needs are information on the distance between the current status and the program's goals. The sources of data are many. Important needs are those the professionals identify as most critical for reaching the program's goals. The needs chosen as priority targets should be directly related to desired student goals and competencies. The next chapter covers planning how to reach the results intended. Remember, _what you plan is what you get._

CHAPTER TEN

Planning for Results

Upon completion of this chapter and its activities, you should be able to demonstrate the following competencies:

- **Know the elements of planning**
- **Know sources for different activities to arrive at a complete plan**
- **Use brainstorming to explore different ways to achieve results**
- **Develop a results plan**

■ *Introduction*

As stated at the end of the last chapter, *what you plan is what you get*. For each competency listed in the Results Agreement, you must have a *plan* for achieving the desired results. A counselor's plan is similar to a teacher's lesson plan, incorporating the same elements that are found in an educational objective:

- The competency to be addressed
- The content of the competency at the specific grade level
- The location where it will be delivered (classroom, office, career center)
- The processes/activities/strategies to be used to achieve the competency
- Timing of when the strategies will be executed and the person responsible for results
- The materials to be used
- The criteria for success and data collection method

■ *Using the Results Planning Form*

Refer to the three sample school results plans on pages 107–109. Each shows a plan for achieving one competency in an elementary, middle school, or high school setting.

Goal Area

The top of the form has a space to indicate the goal area—educational, career, social, or personal—related to the competency being addressed. If the strategy addresses staff, parent, or community targets, it should still tie into a goal for students. In a results-based program, the student remains the primary client, and all student support activities are planned to ensure that students attain the specified goals.

Competency

The columns identify each of the elements in the results plan. The first column identifies the specific competency. This statement should be copied directly from the list of competencies identified in the goals and competencies section of the results-based program (see Chapter 6).

Content

The second column asks you to identify the specific content being taught. For example, the competency might be study skills, but the content will vary by grade level, materials used, and student population. The items listed in this content column will be evaluated to measure whether the competency was attained. Therefore, the more specific and measurable you can make the content, the easier it will be to plan how to evaluate student learning.

Place

Indicating the physical location where the activity will occur allows other counselors and administrators to coordinate their efforts with yours. Many guidance lessons are most appropriately presented to class-size groups, but if several counselors and administrators are planning to utilize a specific instructional area or one teacher's classroom, the location can disrupt the educational environment of the students in that subject.

Processes/Activities

Next comes the step-by-step plan for the process to be used. One planning process involves using 3 x 5 cards to list each step in a team brainstorming session. Using this strategy, everyone thinks of as many things to be done as they can, listing each idea on a separate card. After the brainstorming session, cards are then sequenced into an order to ensure that nothing is forgotten. For example, identifying other curriculum areas with similar objectives could help you find a teacher or class that might have a joint interest in teaching the competency. Scheduling the place and time, collaborating with others who might become involved, locating and/or ordering the materials, reviewing materials, talking with other counselors to get ideas, designing the lesson, and pilot testing it with a small group to find out how effective it will be are all necessary steps in the process to ensure adequate preparation and success. Success, in the end, is found in the details. The more detailed the planning steps are in this column, the more likely it is that the activity will be successful.

Who and When

In this column, specific names are important. The *who* refers to the person responsible for the result as well as the individuals who are participating in the activity. Several adults may be involved in an activity; but one person must retain primary responsibility. This column should not simply say *counselor* or *teacher*. Knowing when the activity will occur and when it will be completed are essential to team planning. This information facilitates the timing of student support results with schoolwide efforts. One obvious example is to plan to teach test-taking strategies before standardized test administration; to do so after students have been tested would miss a critical teaching moment.

Resources

Frequently counselors have difficulty identifying specific resource needs. The plan clearly identifies materials needed and how they are being used. Reflection on the plan helps you identify new materials or resources needed to improve activities for the following year. Information from this column should lead to requests for budgets and materials for the ensuing school year.

Evaluation Criteria

In this column, you must consider ahead of time what level of attainment indicates success for each activity. Is it necessary for 100% of the students to demonstrate 100% of the skills taught, or will a lesser standard be acceptable in some situations? Initially, the criteria for a specific competency may not be as stringent as it will be when it is repeated in future years. In other words, as strategies are tested and perfected, the success rate should get higher. The goal is for all students to attain the competency; however, it may be necessary to accept a minimal level of success for some students. For example, planning and selecting an appropriate educational program to meet one's goals may be a necessary competency for 100% of the students, but 100% of the students may not learn communication skills at the highest level. Minimal competencies in that area may be considered success. Remember, the primary purpose of evaluation is to provide data to help improve the process, not just to prove effectiveness.

Data Collection Methods

Data can be collected in three ways:

1. Students can articulate verbally what they have learned (discussions, answering questions, panel debates, oral exams, etc.).
2. Students can complete written exams, worksheets, written discussion questions, or surveys.
3. Students can demonstrate a skill that someone else can observe and assess (via role-play, in vivo demonstrations, etc.).

The method of data collection must match the activity if students' understanding and skill development are to be measured effectively. Careful planning and sharing of the plan with other team members and administrators facilitates coordination and collaboration. The plan makes the program visible in a concrete format that can be changed as information is gathered on effectiveness, timing, appropriateness, and other factors. The plan also provides a framework for future planning. Through reflection, one can review the steps taken and trace the efficacy of what was contributed and how it was accomplished.

Three sample school plans, with all these elements identified, are included for your use as a guide in completing your own plan.

SAMPLE ELEMENTARY
SCHOOL PLAN

Name: _____

Goal: Education _____ Career _____ Personal/Social __X__ Leisure/Wellness _____

Date: _____

School: _____

Competency	Content	Place	Process/Activities	Who and When	Resources	Evaluation Criteria	Data Collection Methods
Each fifth grade student will demonstrate skills in resolving interpersonal conflicts.	• Reflects content • Reflects feelings • Gives feedback • Arrives at consensus	Classroom during Social Studies	• Develop an outline Definition Examples of Conflict • Pilot test on 3-5 students • Revise • Meet with teachers and arrange time • Meet with principal for approval • Implement -Present definition -Demonstrate examples -Assign students into teams of 3, give each team a simulation -Video each team's presentation -Playback and critique -Complete observation checklist, review with students	Feb 5-12 CDJ	• Overhead • Video camera and tape • Monitor • Handouts for simulation	Each student will correctly demonstrate on videotape, reflection of content and feelings, feedback and facilitating 2 others in arriving at consensus.	• Demonstration on videotape • Critique by counselor and teacher • Observation checklist for self-evaluation

SAMPLE MIDDLE SCHOOL PLAN

Goal: Education _____ Career _____ Personal/Social _____ Leisure/Wellness _____   Date: _____

Competency/ Desired Result	Content	Place	Process/Activities	Who and When	Resources	Evaluation Criteria	Data Collection Methods
Each 8th grade student will describe her/his preferred learning style and matching study skills.	ST = structure Teacher-oriented mastery SF = simulations, type, time and place, groups, processes NT = conceptual futurist independent NF = creative, freedom energy spurts	Guidance Center	• Call students into the Guidance Center in groups of 6-8 • Explain learning style preference • Describe type • Students take and score • Discuss results • Give time and day preference survey • Complete worksheets • Puts info into personal portfolio • Checked by counselor	Mar 3-15 Jan Scott	• Preferential Questionnaire • Handouts • Worksheets • Time of Day Preference Test	List 3 or more learning characteristics of self according to type, time, and place	• Completes assessment and records correctly in Educational Planning Portfolio with preferred learning/study methods. • Validated by counselor and/ or homeroom teacher or advisor

SAMPLE HIGH
SCHOOL PLAN

Name: _____

Goal: _____ Education _____ Career _____ Personal/Social _____ Leisure/Wellness _____

School: _____

Date: _____

Competency/ Desired Result	Content	Place	Process/Activities	Who and When	Resources	Evaluation Criteria	Data Collection Methods
Each student will demonstrate skills in utilizing educational and career software to complete a career and post- high school plan.	• Career interests • Career and college selection • Financial aid qualifications and options	Guidance Center and Computer Center	• Beginning with all grade 12 students, then scheduling each grade level under all are complete • Arrange for college/career software to be networked in computer lab • Work with teacher and other counselors to plan an appropriate schedule • Schedule parents with their students into lab after school • Plan sequence to complete within 2 hrs. for each parent/student • Train 6 parent volunteers to assist in evenings • Upon family completion of process, schedule small group and individual sessions in the Guidance Center	Oct-Feb	• College and career computer software • Computer cards for network • Student portolio • Paper for printouts	• Each student and parent/guardian completes both the career and college search w/ printout. • In case of a mismatch of career and aptitudes, counselor reschedules parent and student for advisement.	• Search info recorded in portfolio. • Counselor reviews portfolio for congruence with current plans and assessed aptitudes. • Review Parent feedback survey.

■ ACTIVITY SET 10.1

Developing a Results Plan

Develop an implementation plan by yourself for one of the results (competencies) stated in your results agreement for which a needs source was identified. The purpose of this exercise is to strengthen your planning skills and to reinforce the use of systems by following a result from mission statement through evaluation process.

A. Please go back to Worksheet 8.1 (page 95), where you wrote a results agreement. Copy a result for which you would like to develop an implementation plan. Write the result/competency in this space:

_____

_____

_____

Separate the result/competency into parts:

Population (for example, seventh graders):_____

_____

Desired competency (for example, time management):   _____

_____

B. Next write what you expect students to learn, i.e. the content. (Example: maintains current homework calendar, describes the importance of time usage, etc.). The content is determined by the characteristics of the selected population, (e.g., developmental level, achievement level, special situations, etc.). For example, study skills for seventh graders have a very different content than those for third graders or eleventh graders; limited English–speaking students require a modification of content to ensure that they will gain the needed competencies; special education students may need the use of specific skills or special techniques to ensure that they succeed.

_____

_____

_____

_____

_____

_____

C. Before completing this part of the activity, think through different processes you might want to use in implementation.

Examples of Processes

- Use individual or group counseling or group guidance.
- Train graduate students from local college or university and/or train parents to work with students.
- Use guidance center activities.
- Provide lunch period "brown bag seminars" (students come to a central location for lunch and bring their own food—counselors provide drinks).
- Use community experts in specific fields or invite retired professionals from the community to meet with individual students (works well with college applications, scholarship search, filling out financial aid forms).
- Train peer counselors and peer tutors.
- Order special materials, videos, posters.

The list of processes is seemingly endless but often rests on the counselors' ability to enlist assistance from others and make others a part of the program. Remember, the plan is not about how the counselor or other student support staff will directly deliver competencies to the student, but rather how the professional will manage the resources available to deliver resources. Once an outsider has participated, that person experiences a feeling of belonging and often will volunteer for future projects.

Form in small groups and use a brainstorming process to gather new alternatives for implementation to get the maximum results. You are encouraged to be creative, to break out of the box, and to utilize the talents of others both in arriving at new ways and in implementing the processes. The brainstorming rules are:

- Contributors will not ask questions.
- Contributions beyond the expected are encouraged.
- No negative responses allowed, such as "that won't work."
- The person presenting the result will take notes and will not make suggestions.

Group members take turns having the group help them by offering different ideas for how to get their stated result. After everyone has had a turn, each person now decides how to implement her or his plan to produce the desired results.

Please list the selected processes and activities in order of how you will achieve your results:

Process and Activities	Who and When
1. _____	_____
2. _____	_____
3. _____	_____
4. _____	_____
5. _____	_____
6. _____	_____
7. _____	_____
8. _____	_____

D. Go back to your list and add the person responsible for each result and when it will be completed.

E. Please list the resources (materials and equipment) you will require to complete the activity:

_____   _____

_____   _____

_____   _____

_____   _____

F. The next step is to establish the evaluation criteria you will use to demonstrate that students have acquired the competencies (knowledge, attitudes, skills) you intend them to achieve. You may want to review the discussion of content earlier in this chapter. Remember, the content forms the criteria of success. For example, seventh grade study skills may include organizational skills, keeping a notebook organized by assignment, and note-taking skills. Evaluation criteria could be a notebook that is neat and accurately kept, with notes on textbook chapters organized by study area.

Results Plan

Name: _____ School _____ Date _____

Goal Area: Education _____ Career _____ Personal/Social _____ Leisure /Wellness _____

Competency/Desired Result	Content	Place	Process/Activities	Who and When	Resources	Evaluation Criteria	Data Collection Methods

_____

_____

_____

_____

_____

G. Indicate how you plan to collect the data. The means of gathering data are usually related to the activities and processes. Consider the three ways to collect data: students can write something (you can read it), they can do something (you can observe them), or they can talk about something (you can listen). All three are appropriate ways to validate student achievement. Using the criteria from the example given, the teacher or assistant could check notebooks weekly and check notes on chapters before each test, and parents could be asked for feedback on the neatness of students' study areas at home.

_____   _____   _____

_____   _____   _____

_____   _____   _____

_____   _____   _____

_____   _____   _____

H. After reviewing and editing this information, transpose it onto Worksheet 10.1 (Results Plan)

Note that the Planning Form provided in this book covers all important steps in the planning process. Counseling practitioners or interns, however, may want to use the planning format used by their district. Most planning formats have similar information elements, but terminology or sequence may differ.

I. Please list all the words you believe should be defined (see Glossary) for others to understand your program results plans. If possible, define them at this time, or you may do the task later.

_____   _____   _____

_____   _____   _____

_____   _____   _____

■ REFLECTION

Please reflect on your thoughts about your involvement in this chapter.

_____

_____

_____

_____

_____

■ SUMMARY

This chapter addresses the process of planning content to achieve your results. The planning process first calls for understanding all the parts of a results plan. The planning format includes identifying the result(s); defining the competencies and listing the competencies students will acquire; deciding where the activity will take place; determining the activities to be used (hopefully, including a pilot study with four to eight students); designating the person(s) accountable for each activity; listing resources that will be needed; stipulating the criteria for success; and describing how data will be collected. In addition, it is important to remember that the primary purpose of evaluation is to improve processes. Therefore, student support professionals are the logical ones to collect and review evaluation data to determine effectiveness and immediately change any process that is not working. Professionals are also advised to use the school district's planning format, if one is available.

The next chapter discusses ways to monitor students' progress in developing the competencies listed in the program results. The school counselor's major accountability is to monitor each student's academic and personal development progress. The counselor, in other words, is the student advocate. Ideally, each and every student will reach the desired results and become a productive citizen.

CHAPTER ELEVEN

Monitoring Student Progress

Upon completion of this chapter and its activities, you should be able to demonstrate the following competencies:

- **Understand the accountability associated with being a student advocate**
- **Explain the different ways advocates can monitor students' behaviors**
- **Plan a student monitoring program that includes parents' involvement**

■ *Introduction*

Monitoring is the process of reviewing data to determine if a student or group of students is demonstrating the desired results as identified in the program goals and related student competencies. Monitoring is one of the most, if not the most, important functions of a counselor in the public schools. This element of responsibility is defined as *advocacy:* the counselor is always an advocate for students as they travel through the educational system. Counselors are expected to consistently monitor students' academic achievements, educational and career planning progress, involvement in extracurricular activities and community service, attendance, and school behaviors. The counselor is responsible for using information to intervene, when necessary, and for confronting any need that is negatively affecting learning and development. Strategies used might include referral to other professionals, individual conferences, conferences with parents and/or teachers, or group or individual counseling.

When available data are reviewed and gaps (needs) are significant, then action must follow to reduce the discrepancies and close the achievement gap. This is the other side of advocacy—taking action. Monitoring and subsequent action take time, but the benefits for students outweigh all other costs.

■ *Monitoring Tools*

Regular ongoing monitoring is achieved through a variety of tools that can become a part of the student support program, such as:

1. *Student education and career planning folders* Students, parents, and teachers use this tool to document and track student progress in attaining competencies related to school success. Student folders are usually stored at school, but they can be taken home periodically for review by parents and returned to school during parent conferences or at the end of the year. These are not the cumulative files kept by the school to maintain legal records.

2. *Parent reference files* Like student folders, this tool facilitates parents' understanding and participation in students' educational endeavors. The parent folder lists not only school-related activities, but also things that can be accomplished at home and in the community to prepare a student for success. Parents can use this file to store school information such as grades, test scores, special awards, and the like.

3. *Student support program monitoring form* A program monitoring form is a checklist that provides the counseling staff with a tool to review its own progress in providing a comprehensive program that has no "holes" or areas of deficit. Monitoring program elements on a periodic basis ensures that all program activities are aligned with the primary mission of the district, the school, and the student support program.

4. *Technology* A variety of technology tools are currently available to monitor student progress. New technology holds even greater promise of efficient and effective monitoring devices. Putting student information (including assignments, grades, and progress-to-date on guidance competencies) on the computer for access by parents and students along with making CDs or "credit cards" with a magnetic strip that can be accessed for monitoring purposes are only a few of the ideas being used by schools.

As technological sophistication grows, the formerly daunting task of ongoing monitoring of student progress promises to become a manageable and very valuable strategy. However, monitoring and reporting progress alone are not adequate to fulfill the student support purpose, which is to ensure that all students are successful. Counselors must be creative in finding the means to assist students in attaining the competencies they need to become productive adults. Perhaps the most valuable ally in this endeavor is the parent. Finding ways to involve parents in the monitoring process greatly increases the possibility of success.

■ ACTIVITY SET 11.1

Areas to Be Monitored and Sources of Data

In identifying areas that should be monitored, it is also necessary to determine sources of data, including the following: academic achievement, educational and career development competencies, attendance, extracurricular activities, community services, conflict-based referrals, and school site interpersonal behaviors.

A. In the first column, list areas of student behaviors you believe should be monitored. (Example: student academic achievement = grades, test scores, course completion, challenging courses taken, scholarship qualifications.)

Monitored Student Behaviors	Sources of Data
_____	_____
_____	_____
_____	_____
_____	_____
_____	_____
_____	_____

B. In a small group, brainstorm other sources of student performance that can be monitored to facilitate reaching the goals and student competencies of both the school and the student support program. (Example: service to school and community = membership in school clubs, community organization, community service hours, volunteer activities.)

Other Areas of Student Performance	Sources of Data
_____	_____
_____	_____
_____	_____
_____	_____

_____   _____

_____   _____

                                _____

_____   _____

C. Turn to Worksheet 11.1 (What Gets Monitored Gets Done), on page 121.
Complete the following:

1. In columns 1 and 2, identify area/competency/behaviors for specific
   grades and enter them in the appropriate places.

2. In columns 3 and 4, enter the intervention strategies you will use, including
   when and how.

3. In columns 5 and 6, write in the success indicators and how you will collect
   and record the data.

4. After completing the worksheet, reflect here on the processes of student
   advocacy, on monitoring, and on intervening when appropriate.

_____

_____

_____

_____

_____

What Gets Monitored Gets Done

Grade	Area/Competency/Behavior	When	Intervention Strategies	Success Indicators	How Recorded

D. Parents also have responsibility for monitoring their student's educational progress. Many if not most, however, require help in knowing the how and what of the process. This is the student support team's contribution to families—to instruct parents on how to monitor their children's educational progress and identify the tools and data available to parents. This information may be in the school's handbook for students and parents. The following table shows some examples. You can add to the list.

PARENTAL MONITORING

What	How
1. Report cards	Maintain an ongoing record of the student's progress, noting strengths.
2. Learning rituals in the home	Make sure that the student maintains a regular scheduled time to study, at least 4 days a week.
3. Counselor/teacher conference	Review annually the updated printout on the student's plans, including results of educational and career computer searches.
4.	
5.	
6.	

■ *Using the School Profile as a Resource for Monitoring Students' Achievement*

The current school profile information is an excellent source of data for monitoring students' educational progress. The reported profile information depends on the school's or school district's priorities. The profile also serves as the basis for the school's *evaluation portfolio*, a document that presents overall school (and student support) program results.

What the School Profile Does

- Documents efforts on results achievement
- Provides ready, necessary information for data-based decision making
- Reflects progress toward mission and goal achievement
- Allows for data use as a guide in continual program improvement
- Shows accountability and communication
- Invites reflection and participation

What the School Profile Contains

- Student learning: standardized test scores, criterion reference data, teacher observations, authentic assessment data
- Demographics: enrollment, gender, ethnicity, attendance, dropout, grade levels, languages
- School processes: description of school programs and processes
- Perceptions: of learning environments, values, beliefs, attitudes, observations

How You Can Use the Information

The information in the school profile is extremely valuable for all student support personnel. For example, achievement by subject can be broken down by gender, ethnicity, referrals, and many other available variables. It becomes the *responsibility of the counselor* to request specific data that can be used to reduce the disparities in achievement and involvement, where and when appropriate.

■ *Impact of the Comprehensive Results-Based Student Support Program*

Collecting and analyzing data on a multiyear basis allows trend analysis of the impact of the comprehensive results-based student support program. The forms provided in Activity Set 11.2 were designed to begin the collection and use of data that demonstrates student support contributions to the educational program in terms of impact on specific outcomes.

■ ACTIVITY SET 11.2

Data Collection and Analysis over Four Years

Using Worksheet 11.2 (Impact of the Comprehensive Results-Based Student Support Program) on page 125, you are encouraged to fill in the information, add other available data, maintain the data to see what impact you have made, and to reflect on what elements of the school community you can impact. Add additional items that provide data on program impact.

Impact of the Comprehensive
Results-Based Student Support Program

School _____

Principal / Counselor / Psychologist / Nurse _____

School Year _____

Date _____

	Year 1	Year 2	Year 3	Year 4
1.0 School Climate:				
1.1 Attendance				
Truancies				
Excused Absences				
Unexcused Absences				
Other				
1.2 Discipline Year				
Classroom Referrals				
Outside of Classroom Referrals				
Other				
1.3 Vandalism				
Incidents				
Costs				
Other				

	Year 1	Year 2	Year 3	Year 4
1.4 Parent Involvement				
Scheduled Conferences				
Unscheduled Conferences				
*Co-Support				
*Co-Learning				
*Co-Teaching				
*Co-Decision Making				
Other				
1.5 Student Involvement				
SAT/ACT Prep				
Study Skills Sessions				
Community Service				
College Applications				
Financial Aid Applications				
Career Selection & Planning				
Student Government				
Sports				
Portfolio Development				
Extracurricular Activities				
Other				

	Year 1	Year 2	Year 3	Year 4
2.0 Academic Achievement:				
2.1 SAT Scores				
Verbal Composite				
Math				
2.2 ACT				
Verbal				
Math				
2.3 State Standardized Tests				
Reading				
Language				
Math				
Other				
2.3 GPA (Use Current Data Provided by the System				
% Passing				
% Passing Math by Grade				
% Passing Science by Grade				
2.4 Other				
Advanced Placement				
International Baccalaureate				
Community College Classes				
SAT 9				

*Examples

Co-support: Parents and educators agree on a plan for the student, both follow through, monitor, and reverse if needed

Co-learning: Parent workshops and parent/educator workshops taught by experts in an area, e.g. bullying, learning styles, etc.

Co-teaching: Parents assist in teaching in areas of expertise, e.g., career days, college days, subject areas, etc.

Co-decision making: Parents and counselors make collaborative decisions on student placement, activities, monitoring schedules, long-range plans.

■ REFLECTION

Please post your reflections about the chapter on monitoring.

_____

_____

_____

_____

_____

■ SUMMARY

This chapter reviews the primary accountability of a school counselor—being the students' advocate (Martin & House, 2003). The process of advocacy is accomplished through monitoring students' academic and personal development, and intervening when deficiencies are noted. There are numerous sources of data available for review, and most are available without for the need for further data processing. This chapter includes a review of school profile information as well as methods for locating data and who should be involved. More important, as a result of work done by the Education Trust (2003), school counselors are advised to take a leadership role in using available data as a means to change existing problems and confront the need to close the gap for underachieving youth.

CHAPTER TWELVE

Using Calendars for Program Success

Upon completion of this chapter and its activities, you should be able to demonstrate the following competencies:

- **Know the importance of keeping a detailed calendar of student support program activities**
- **Understand how calendars contribute to program visibility**
- **Develop a master calendar and disseminate it effectively**

■ *Introduction*

In traditional programs, school counselors complain that they have little time for planned guidance program activities because they are assigned too many duties peripheral to their job and because so many crises occur. One must remember that schools are places where students spend much of their time and that each childhood and adolescent stage is rife with normal developmental crises. Learning to address and solve crises is a major task of youth. Counselors have traditionally treated these predictable crises as times to help students solve their problems. The results-based approach is predicated on a philosophy that teaching students problem-solving skills will have longer lasting effects than simply helping them solve specific problems on an as needed basis.

■ *Advantages of the Student Support Program Calendar*

In describing their daily schedules, counselors traditionally complain that as soon as they enter school premises, the day "happens to them." A calendar, however, helps the counselor "happen to the day." A schedule filled with referrals of behavioral problem students or feuding students or students dropping in with hopes that someone else will resolve their problems makes it hard to plan the day or the week or the year. Hall and lunchroom duty, scheduling classes, and other tasks that any less trained staff member could accomplish are greatly reduced when counselors develop a scheduled calendar linked to producing student results.

Throughout this workbook, we have emphasized the importance of planning an efficient and effective program and then reporting it in a highly visible manner. In this way school counselors educate the entire school community about the nature of their job. Comprehensive and thorough planning allows school counselors to "capture" pieces of their time and, through results reporting, assure the administration and faculty that program implementation is the best use of professional time.

Reporting after the fact does not adequately inform the rest of the school about the appropriate use of a school counselor's time. A calendar, well planned and disseminated in such a way that everyone knows the counselor's availability, goes a long way toward making time available for all of the important activities as well as informing school staff when particular referrals are appropriate. Few would consider simply walking into a classroom and taking the teacher out to do a mundane, nonteaching task during class time. A well-organized calendar for the school counseling office can accomplish a similar reorientation toward the importance of counseling.

If teachers and administrators know when and which counselors are available and the important tasks they are undertaking when they are *not* available, they are more likely to respect those plans and work with counselors. In addition, a calendar makes it clear when counselors are going to be working with teachers, classes, and target student populations in preplanned and productive ways. It not only informs others of the efficient and effective ways that the counselor serves the school community and shows the breadth of tasks undertaken, it also provides those who want to refer students, information on specific times when crisis intervention counseling is available. Frustration is lessened and the whole staff begins to understand and appreciate the well-organized student support team.

■ *The Yearly Calendar*

The consistent use and maintenance of an annual program calendar, coordinated with the school calendar, facilitates staff, parent, student, and community involvement as partners in students' educational endeavors and as advocates for student support functions. In addition, the calendar establishes a schedule for student support activities. As the program grows and multiple activities are developed, a calendar reflects the important benefits that the student support program provides for students, parents, teachers, and administrators.

Developing a program calendar for the entire school year is a way to identify each program commitment—the date and day, the nature of the activity, the scheduled time, and the targeted audience. It is sometimes helpful to highlight in different colors specific aspects of the calendar (e.g., grade levels, domains, identified populations such as ESL or college-bound students) and curriculum specialties, such as school-to-career. Events and activities designed for all students can also be highlighted in a specific identifiable color. Ideally, the program calendar should be located in several prominent places such as the department bulletin board, school or student bulletin boards, classroom bulletin boards, administrative offices, parent center, career center, student store, and other sites used to communicate school events. It may also be submitted to the local newspaper and the student newspaper to increase the program's visibility.

The student support calendar might include relevant school activities—other than those provided by the student support program—that affect the family, such as back-to-school nights, open houses, PTA meetings, dates when standardized tests are scheduled, parent-student-teacher conferences, planned guidance classroom units, career or college nights, evening meetings for reviewing study skills, or other opportunities provided through the school and the community.

Many schools provide a yearly schedule of school activities that can be coordinated with student support events, including all relevant dates and times noted on the student support calendar. Effective use of the student support program calendar does the following:

- Increases the visibility of student support program and other related educational activities

- Provides focus on events/activities of value to students, parents, and staff

- Increases communication within the school and home about schedules and program activities

- Facilitates student, family, department, and school planning for future important student support functions

- Establishes an organizational pattern of highlighting and valuing student support opportunities

- Reinforces the importance of student participation in student support-related activities

The Monthly Calendar

The monthly calendar is maintained and circulated to highlight specific activities and events for each month occurring throughout the school year and during the summer. The monthly calendar should be printed in a distinctive color and distributed to each teacher for classroom bulletin boards before the beginning of each month. It should include a reminder to teachers that they are invited to participate and to encourage student participation or observance of upcoming events such as college application dates, SAT deadline dates, study skills workshops, and scheduled career and/or college planning for students and their parents. The calendar should be mailed to parents as well.

A well-developed monthly calendar that is complete, timely, and color-ful can be a powerful public relations booster. Time and careful thought should be given to the consistency in timing and methods of distribution and to the calendar's format and attractiveness of design, color, and detail. An effective calendar invites others to acknowledge and participate in student support program activities.

A sample monthly calendar below is presented to encourage your thinking about how your school calendar can promote the student support program.

SAMPLE CALENDAR
STUDENT SUPPORT PROGRAM: NOVEMBER 2006

MONDAY	TUESDAY	WEDNESDAY	THURSDAY	FRIDAY
		(1) Personal/Social: Conflict Resolution—U.S. Hist per. 5, 6 6:00–9:00* Counselor appts. available—call ahead	(2) Career Planning Gr. 9—Social Studies classes per. 2, 3	(3) Career Planning Gr. 9—Social Studies classes per. 2, 3
(6) Student Support Center visit—Gr. 9 Soc Studies—per. 2, 3 5:00 m.— New Student Orientation	(7) Sr. transcript requests due for college submission Sr. Seminar[†] 5:00 m.—ESL Orientation	(8) Sr. mtgs.— Review college applications, +post–H.S. plans 6:00–9:00* Counselor appts. available in Student Support Center	(9) Sr. mtgs.— Review college applications + post–H.S. plans	(10) Sr. mtgs.— Review college applications + Post–H.S. plans
(13) Career Day—Gr. 9–10 in Guid. Center, all periods—Engl. classes	(14) Sr. Seminar[†]	(15) 6:00–9:00* Counselor appts. available in Student Support Center	(16) Gr. 12 Engl. classes—review study skills, Cornell note taking	(17) Guid. Center visits—Gr. 11, Sci. classes—to update portfolios
(20) Career Day—Gr. 11–12 in Student Support Center, all periods—Engl. classes	(21) Sr. Seminar[†]	(22) No Evening Appts.	(23) THANKSGIVING HOLIDAY	(24) THANKSGIVING HOLIDAY
(27) Career Night—Students, Staff, Parents invited	(28) Sr. Seminar[†]	(29) No Evening Appts.	(30) 6:30: Parent Night—Preparing your student for college	

* Seniors: Brownbag seminars every Tues. at lunch in Guidance Center: Preparing for College: What should you know? For information or to make an appointment, call the Guidance Center at 000-123-4567 or email: sjohnso4@cox.net

[†] For information or to make an appointment, call the Guidance Center, 000-123-4567 or email: sjohnso4@cox.net

■ ACTIVITY SET 12.1

Planning a Student Support Program Calendar

A. In a small group, discuss the following considerations:

1. What nonnegotiable events and dates should be included in planning a student support program calendar? For example, consider yearly events that are scheduled by the district, colleges, and community (student registration, standardized testing, college application deadlines, student course selection, SAT/ACT/AP testing, open house, etc.).

_____

_____

_____

_____

_____

_____

_____

_____

2. Develop a timeline for producing the calendar. Who will post notices? What are the deadline dates to ensure that it can be completed and distributed in a timely manner each month?

_____

_____

_____

_____

_____

3. Brainstorm strategies that can be used to make your student support program calendar unique and noticed. Consider a unique color (fluorescent pink, orange, purple) and a "surround," that is, develop a distinctive bulletin board design and post the monthly calendar regularly as part of that bulletin board. Adopt a logo or format that is different from other announcements sent out from the school. Brainstorm ideas that seem workable for you.

_____

_____

_____

_____

_____

4. To whom will the calendar be distributed (classroom bulletin boards, parents, local newspaper, principal's newsletter, student support office, main office, district office, etc.)?

_____

_____

_____

_____

B. What other ideas do you have for promoting, making visible, and building public relations for the student support program? Make a list.

_____

_____

_____

_____

_____

_____

_____

_____

_____

C. Using Worksheet 12.1, which follows page 143, design a monthly calendar of events at a fictitious elementary, middle, or high school.

▪ REFLECTION

Please post your reflections on the use of student support program calendars.

_____

_____

_____

_____

_____

▪ SUMMARY

This chapter has been constructed to emphasize the importance of maintaining a calendar for student support program activities on a yearly, weekly, and monthly basis. The calendar can be used to make the program visible to all parties affected by the program, including teachers, parents, community members, and administrators. Where and how the calendar is disseminated affects the impact it can have. When it is widely distributed, the calendar encourages voluntary participation in planned activities, facilitates advance planning for parents and others who would like to participate in activities such as college and career nights, and advertises the range of contributions made by the student support program. The next chapter addresses the advantages of having a student support program advisory council.

School _____

Student Support Program Calendar for the Month of _____

Monday	Tuesday	Wednesday	Thursday	Friday

CHAPTER THIRTEEN

Student Support Advisory Councils

Upon completion of this chapter and its activities, you should be able to demonstrate the following competencies:

- **Describe the advantages of having a student support advisory council**
- **Identify the membership, including representative populations, organizations, and other members of the school community**
- **Identify the major functions of the council**
- **Create a council and plan meetings and agendas**

■ *Introduction*

The U.S. Constitution guarantees each citizen the right to an education. Community control over the educational process has been maintained through school boards of education. Elected or appointed school board members have achieved this honor because their values are represent those of the community. In this way, a community's values are transmitted through the educational curriculum to that community's youth. Schools thus represent what local adult community members value for their youth.

Large school systems representing large populations present a more complicated situation for community input than small districts because school board members represent and make decisions for a large and usually more diverse body of citizens. School systems with 30 or more schools probably have more difficulty attempting to represent communal values than do school systems with 10 to 15 schools. Large communities have subpopulations with specific needs. Therefore, where a system has two or more secondary schools, the needs of each school population might be different.

Professional educators are paid specialists charged with developing educational goals, curriculum, and processes that perpetuate the values of a local community. Therefore, at the county, district, and school-building level, parent advisory groups have been established to advise administrators and school board members on what they believe educational goals should be and, subsequently, what curriculum content should be offered to their students. *A community or parent advisory group is an appointed group of citizens who are charged with two objectives: (1) auditing educational goals and (2) recommending priorities.* Specifically, at the school building level, parent/community advisory groups can be an asset to educators by voicing concerns, prioritizing educational goals, and recommending various actions.

The purpose of this chapter is to suggest ways to use advisory groups, specifically student support advisory councils. We will present ideas about forming student support advisory councils at the district and local school level, including a meeting schedule with possible agendas, auxiliary functions, and evaluation strategies. These materials can be used as guidelines in developing community involvement and community support for the student support program.

Now more than ever before, with the changing role of student support programs, student support professionals need involvement and input from the school community. Student support staff have moved from the academic advisor stage through the humanistic individual and group counseling era to our present status of potential extinction because of shortages of funds, lack of support, and lack of evidence of our contributions. Professional journals suggest that our present mode of dealing with one student at a time on a crisis or reactive basis must be reexamined. Further, it is abundantly clear that student support programs must be based on clearly stated, visible goals and related competencies with processes designed to assist each student.

■ *Forming a Student Support Advisory Council (SSAC)*

Student support programs reflect student needs and community values. Further, the student support program goals and student competencies are designed by student support personnel and are supported by needs data and professional expertise related to developmental stages of learning, career development, interpersonal skills, and personal growth. Although professionals design the program, *the responsibility of validating the goals and student competencies must be delegated to students and community members.* One of the most efficient means of getting this validation is to form and use a student support advisory council (SSAC). It is the student support department's responsibility to allocate energy and resources to establishing an SSAC.

Although an advisory council may seem like a lot of work, there are many advantages to investing in this activity. First, the ties that are built across the community enrich the types of curricula developed as the needs, interests, and talents of students, parents, administration, teachers, and the business community are brought to bear in open discussion. Second, the credibility of the student support program is bolstered by ensuring that it takes into account the perspective of the whole community.

Program visibility provided by the SSAC offers an avenue for encouraging families and the community to participate in program activities, encourage student participation, and make program activities a planned and expected part of the school calendar. Visibility may prove to be the most important asset the student support program develops. Suggested members of the advisory council include individuals from the community at large, school administrators, and faculty. The SSAC chair should be a person with skills in planning and conducting meetings, proven group guidance skills, and demonstrate consistently positive attitudes toward others. A counselor or other student support team member should serve on the committee as a facilitator. The amount of time the facilitator can expect to allocate to this responsibility will depend upon the number of contributions SSAC members make.

The advisory council provides feedback to student support program efforts and receives regular reports that include positive student results, which help build a supportive attitude toward school counselors and the student support team. When advisory council representatives from the school district office, administration, or school board regularly see dramatic results from the efforts of school counselors, they become advocates for the program and support requests for resources and budget. Credible, effective, high-profile student support teams are one of the most important assets of the school community. There is much incentive for the extra effort it takes to develop and maintain a student support program advisory council.

Auxiliary Functions of the SSAC

The quantity and quality of contributions depend upon the members of the SSAC and their interests and commitment to the program. Although it is not the council's purpose to have members assist in the program, SSAC members sometimes volunteer to help in registration and program-changing activities; some volunteer to acquire needed guest speakers; others volunteer to assemble scholarship booklets. Some SSAC members become peer counselors or volunteer to host coffee klatches and make presentations to local community groups and school boards. Members should not be expected to go beyond their specified responsibilities to audit the program and make recommendations. However, volunteer activities by council members that build a sense of understanding and support for the program goals are usually welcomed by student support team members. Specific, official SSAC activities will be addressed later in this section.

Steps in Establishing a School SSAC

Counselors and others who are considering forming an SSAC may want to adopt their own planning format based on the following steps.

1. Developing and implementing a results-based student support program comes first. The program philosophy, goals, competencies, management system, results agreements, and results plans are completed and audited by the principal and coordinator/supervisor of the student support program.

2. The student support department decides to form a student support advisory council. One team member volunteers (or is selected) to be the SSAC facilitator.

3. The facilitating team member develops a plan that includes the SSAC's purpose, suggested membership, and tentative meeting dates with proposed agendas. (The SSAC can be a separate school committee or can be a subcommittee of an existing SAC, PTA, or PTSA.)

4. The SSAC plan is reviewed by the other student support staff members and is modified where appropriate.

■ *Managing the School SSAC*

The Student Support Advisory Council can be an efficient and effective tool when it is managed with clear purpose and direction.

Purpose

The purpose of a student support advisory council is to audit goals and student competencies and to make recommendations on priorities. The facilitator with the responsibility of managing the SSAC must make sure that each member understands this purpose. The responsibility for designing and implementing processes rests with the school's student support staff. If this distinction is unclear, there might be a tendency to discuss and approve or evaluate processes, thus violating the freedom and creativity of the counselors. The student support staff and the student support advisory council must both understand and respect the responsibilities and constraints of each group. This respect creates a harmonious and supportive atmosphere where innovation is encouraged.

Auditing the Program

The auditing and recommending function should address all elements of the results-based student support program. Specifically the SSAC is responsible for ensuring that the stated mission, goals, and competencies are accurate reflections of the aspirations of the students, parents, and broader school community. The student support advisory council members can provide valuable input ensuring that all activities and resources focus on school and community priorities. The composition of the SSAC should be varied enough to allow for reviews of program elements from each representative group in the community. Recommendations are made to the school administrator or school board members and should address only the desired results of the program, not the activities used to reach results.

Individual Concerns

The facilitator should realize that the council members come to the council for different reasons. Some may accept the position because they want to learn more about the program, others because they have preconceptions of what is good and what should be changed. It is the facilitator's responsibility to meet with members individually to learn their concerns, ideas, and expectations. With this knowledge, the facilitator with group skills can help accomplish the SSAC's purposes as well as address individual expectations.

Processes

The student support department is responsible for designing and implementing the processes (means) to achieve the desired results. In this area the freedom and creativity of the counselors is paramount. The atmosphere should be one where innovation is encouraged but results and cost effectiveness are equally important. Scrutiny of student results is essential to continual improvement of the program.

School Observation

After purpose and processes have been explained and questions answered, it is time to arrange for all SSAC members collectively, in small groups, or individually to visit the school (by appointment) to see the student support program in process. A guide on what to look for might include the following:

- How inviting is the student support office? Are students and parents welcomed when they enter the office?
- Are the offices neat and well organized? Are there posters and other colorful signs related to student interests?
- Is a clear method in place to access services and materials?
- Is there a guidance center with resource materials available to students and parents? Is the guidance center welcoming? Is there a process for checking out materials such as college catalogs and scholarship materials? Are there free materials for students to take home and read?
- Is the guidance center utilized by students during the day, during lunch periods, and before and after school?
- Do staff members know students by name? Do they attempt to remember students' names?
- Is the guidance office clearly marked and easy to locate?
- Is there a parent center or area within the guidance center with educational and guidance materials for parents? Is a computer and software program for college/career planning available for parents?
- Is someone present to help with appointments and to know schedules for staff members (school psychologist, social worker, etc.) who may not be on campus every day?
- How do staff members appear to interact with other faculty members, with clerical staff, with administrators?
- Is a calendar posted with guidance activities listed?

Verbal Needs Assessment

A verbal needs assessment is important for effective functioning of the SSAC. After visiting the school, the SSAC should respond if it feels any area it observed was lacking. The facilitator or secretary records responses. This list might be used to encourage SSAC members to make their own contributions. For example, in one school several SSAC members wanted more emphasis placed on counseling college-bound students. Since they understood the constraints of a large counselor-student ratio and a small number of students who probably would benefit, they offered their assistance. They agreed to work with a counselor on a project to create a college handbook including requirements and financial aids, to be distributed to each student who had declared an interest in going on to an institution of higher education.

Public Relations

When the student support advisory council is visible to the school administration and community, its members often become student support program experts in their neighborhood. Sometimes community members will express concerns to individual SSAC members that they won't communicate to school professionals. Council members are able to buffer complaints from the community based upon misinformation or lack of knowledge about what is actually happening. Their role as community liaison is informal and occurs slowly as SSAC members experience growing involvement in and support for the student support program. Although this function may not be explicitly encouraged, it is perhaps one of the most positive public relations contacts a student support department can develop.

Recognition

The counseling staff is encouraged to host the final council meeting or a special meeting at a breakfast or luncheon. During this activity, the counseling staff needs to express its appreciation for the amount of effort contributed by each member and the SSAC as a whole. Building-level administrators should be invited as well as a district-level representative, and a representative from a local newspaper should be invited and encouraged to acknowledge publicly the SSAC's contributions to the local community.

Reporting

Plans need to be completed for submitting the final report to the district SSAC. It is most effective if one or more local SSAC members presents the report. If this is not possible, the final report should be presented to the district SSAC with copies distributed at the local school for reporting purposes. The SSAC should also make a presentation to the school staff and/or to the parent-teacher organization.

Annual Report

Each local school SSAC gives an annual report to the district SSAC in June. In preparing the annual report, the council chair and the facilitator might want to consider a short and concise format that includes the following:

- SSAC membership and goals
- Commendations and recommendations
- Appendices (copy of program document, names of student support team members, student support budget, SSAC activities for the year)

Selecting Local School SSAC Members

Size and representation are critical issues in the ultimate effectiveness of the council.

Council Size

The effectiveness of the student support advisory council is dependent upon two important factors: group size and group composition. Ideally, council membership should be maintained at 10 to 15 members. A group larger than 15 becomes cumbersome, and a group of less than 10 puts too much responsibility on each person in time necessary to accomplish council tasks. Also, the council should be large enough to include participants from a comprehensive cross-section of community, school, and student membership.

Population Concerns

Although it may be easier to find willing participants from a single segment of the community, this practice should be avoided. For example, college-oriented parents may have the time for, and interest in, school-related committees. However, if the majority of the SSAC members represent any one segment of the community, student support staff may find goal priorities skewed toward meeting the needs of one type of student, such as college/university-bound students, at the expense of other populations.

Parent and Community Representation

A balanced representation of community subpopulations is necessary to assure that student support goals will be prioritized to help all students. Balancing considerations should include geographical locations, religious representation, ethnic representation, economic levels, occupational levels, and gender representation.

Teacher Representation

It is equally important to include teachers from the school as members of the SSAC. Whenever possible, a teacher from an academic area and a teacher from a vocational area should be recruited. The teachers add the perspective of what teachers need and want in guidance results for students. They also become advocates of student support contributions and concerns.

Student Representation

Student members give yet another perspective in setting priorities. A high school SSAC should have one student member representing grades 9–10 and one student member representing grades 11–12. Their input will support developmentally derived student results and will also serve as a sounding board for ideas and recommendations made by council members. It is sometimes difficult to maintain the interest and involvement of middle school and elementary students, but some younger students have served on these councils and have been very helpful.

Administrative Representation

An optional representative is a school and/or district administrator. Many times the administrator will opt to attend only meetings where her/his direct input is requested. This is often because of a very busy schedule and/or a reluctance to impose administrative concerns on the priority setting of guidance goals. If the administrator does attend, it is crucial that she/he understands that her/his participation is desired as a member but not as the leader of the group.

Other Representation

Other representatives selected from service groups, business clubs, professional associations, school district personnel, and/or the district school board will further ensure balanced representation on the council.

Recruitment Methods

Recruitment can be done by preselecting, asking for volunteers at large group meetings such as back-to-school nights, letters to all or a random sample of parents, announcements to service club presidents, and/or recommendations from school staff. Whatever method is used, it is recommended that each person be contacted by phone and by a personal letter thanking her/him for volunteering to assist. As part of the recruitment materials it is important to stipulate the extent of commitment requested, including number of meetings, proposed dates and times, and other responsibilities. Participants are more willing to make commitments when there are clear parameters from the beginning.

Purpose

Advisory groups for the school system, school, or individual departments share the same basic purposes: (1) to audit goals, plans, and evaluative data, and (2) to recommend priorities to appropriate authorities. The student support advisory council is a departmental advisory group in which members jointly share a special interest in the student support functions of the school. Because of this special interest, the SSAC might be utilized in a number of auxiliary ways and might be expected to become an adjunct to the student support department. However, it is important that the SSAC fulfills its primary functions of auditing and recommending before any SSAC member becomes involved in other student support-related activities.

■ *District Student Support Advisory Council*

The size of a district may determine the membership and purpose of the District Advisory Council.

Council Size

The district SSAC is larger than the school-based council because it provides representation from a wide range of populations including all schools, district-level personnel, community, and others.

Membership

Although similar in nature to local school SSACs, the district SSAC should be representative of the total school system community. Members of the council should include representatives from:

- Student body (2–3 members)
- Parents from each school level (elementary, middle/junior, and senior high) and, if necessary, from each of the local regional areas

- A sampling of district community groups and organizations
- Board of Education and the district administration staff
- All segments of the community (socioeconomic groups, ethnic/racial groups, religious representation, occupational levels, and male/female representation)

In addition, the council should include the supervisor of student support programs and the director of pupil services. (Membership should be on a rotating basis so that there is never a time when all committee members are new.)

Purpose

Advisory groups for the school system, school, or individual departments share the same basic purposes: (1) to audit goals, plans, and evaluative data, and (2) to recommend priorities. In addition, the district SSAC assumes responsibility for

- Monitoring the progress of local school student support programs.
- Reviewing end-of-year reports from local school student support programs.
- Preparing a composite end-of-year report of local school student support programs for the school board.
- Presenting an end-of-year report with recommendations and testifying to school boards and district councils on issues germane to student support program.

Meetings

The district SSAC will meet quarterly to monitor the progress of local school SSACs. These meetings can be presented as workshops and should include representatives from local school SSACs. Because of the size of the district SSAC and the extent of monitoring that may need to be addressed (depending upon the number of schools), it may be advantageous for the SSAC to subdivide into special interest groups based upon school grade levels (elementary, middle/junior, and senior high); regional areas; or special interests (i.e., career planning). At the initial district SSAC general meeting, the superintendent or her/his designee should give greetings to the council. Each local school SSAC should provide the district SSAC with a copy of its minutes not later than one month after each meeting.

In addition to quarterly meetings (more often if necessary), two workshops for local committee members (fall and spring) can be held to in-service participants on

- Student support program elements.
- Administrative procedures.
- Effective ways of auditing student support departments' program (philosophies, goals, competencies, plans, etc.).
- Other pertinent matters.

School Visitations

A member (or members) of the district SSAC should regularly visit one or more of the meetings held by the local school SSAC. At these meetings, the district SSAC representative can act as a resource to relay needed information from the district SSAC. Moreover, this person may monitor the meeting to ascertain its effectiveness, provide direction where needed, and coordinate efforts between the committees.

Recognition

During the final meeting of the year, local school SSAC members should be recognized for their contributions to the local school student support departments. Keeping in mind that some committees may be more active than others, opportunities should be provided to highlight the accomplishments of the various committees. It is suggested that the superintendent or her/his designee, local school administrators, and board of education members be invited to this meeting.

Sample District SSAC Calendar

Calendar of Quarterly Meetings

First Meeting: General District SSAC membership meeting. At the meeting, the chair, co-chair, and secretary are elected. The supervisor or director of student support acts as an adjunct member. An agenda for the year is also set at this meeting. In subsequent years, the agenda for the next year will be set at the last meeting of the previous year.

Second Meeting: Joint meeting with representatives from each local SSAC to be held at a central location. Audit progress of establishment of local school SSACs and make recommendations where necessary.

Third Meeting: Joint meeting with representatives from each local SSAC to discuss progress of local councils and constraints experienced by the local school councils. Distribution of forms for end-of-year reports. This meeting could also include representatives from SSACs in adjoining districts (as a sharing session).

Fourth Meeting: Joint meeting to plan for next school year. Discussion of end-of-year reports. The district SSAC chair presents to the Board of Education the results of the program auditing, with recommendations for priorities.

Sample Meeting Agendas for Local or District-Level Advisory Councils

Meeting 1: Make introductions; provide orientation; establish schedule of meetings; selection of chair, co-chair, and secretary; distribute and discuss SSAC purposes; determine needed resources and supplies; set agenda for the year and establish time commitment; and present overview and explanation of student support program, including competencies from each school.

Meeting 2: Review minutes of last meeting; review status of student support program (by facilitators); discuss student support program; prioritize needs based upon stated program competencies; audit student support program results; and set schedule for school visitations.

Meeting 3: Review minutes of last meeting; discuss results of school visitations; establish SSAC contributions that can facilitate attainment of student support outcomes; formulate plans inclusive of dates; and determine evaluation data for end-of-year report.

Meeting 4: Review minutes of last meeting; review, prepare, and approve annual report for the Board of Education; and set next meeting agenda. Develop agenda of future meetings, based upon the expressed needs of the SSAC. Remind the facilitator that at each meeting the SSAC should audit goals, competencies, related processes, and evaluative data. Commend, and make recommendations on, selected aspects of the program. Remember that data for the end-of-year report must be compiled during these meetings.

■ **ACTIVITY SET 13.1**

These activities will help you apply the knowledge gained in this chapter to developing practical plans for a student support advisory council in a specific setting.

A. Role-play situations. After each of the following scenarios, describe what you would do in such a situation.

1. The SSAC decides upon priorities that are in conflict with the interests of one or more of the student support staff.

_____

_____

_____

_____

2. The SSAC has several representatives with a strong bias in one direction who are attempting to control the total group. The chair attends meetings but fails to provide adequate leadership.

_____

_____

_____

_____

3. The SSAC members have fallen into a pattern of spending much of the meeting time discussing problems they see occurring with their own children.

_____

_____

_____

_____

4. The SSAC begins to assume roles and functions that are inappropriate to the goals of the group.

_____

_____

_____

_____

5. The general tone of SSAC meetings is, "The problems of the younger generation are . . ."

_____

_____

_____

B. Answer the following questions. Be as specific as you can. Name names, cite organizations, set dates for each phase to be completed, and note additional information needed to complete this task.

1. What are the purpose and functions of a student support advisory council?

_____

_____

_____

_____

2. Describe the advantages a student support advisory council can provide for your program.

_____

_____

_____

_____

3. List the selection criteria you will use to choose individual SSAC members.

_____

_____

_____

_____

_____

4. What specific groups are to be represented and what individuals will be considered?

_____

_____

_____

_____

5. What recruitment methods will you employ to assure necessary representation?

_____

_____

_____

_____

6. Set a timeline of tasks to be completed as part of the recruitment and indicate who will be responsible for each task.

Task	Completion Date	Task Completed By

7. Prepare a plan to provide the in-service training that SSAC members will need to begin their assigned tasks.

_____

_____

_____

_____

8. Prepare a plan to provide any additional training needed for the chair.

_____

_____

_____

_____

9. Set a timeline of tasks to be completed for the training component and the person responsible for each task.

Task	Completion Date	Task Completed By

C. Prepare sample agendas for the first three meetings and identify the major concerns for each meeting planned.

MEETING	AGENDA	MAJOR CONCERNS
1.		
2.		
3.		

D. Worksheet 13.1 provides a record of SSAC activities that can be completed now for practice or saved for later use on site by the counselor-in-training intern or the counseling graduate.

■ REFLECTION

Please post your reflections on the use of a Student Support Advisory Council.

_____

_____

_____

_____

_____

_____

_____

Sample Activity Record

STUDENT SUPPORT ADVISORY COUNCIL

School: _____ Area: _____ Date: _____

Person Reporting: _____

(Name) (Title/Category)

COUNCIL INFORMATION

1. List members and their categories (Parent, Student, etc.):

Member Name	Category
1.	
2.	
3.	
4.	
5.	

Total members: _____

2. Give dates of committee meetings:

_____

_____

_____

_____

3. Give names and categories of people attending district workshops.

Fall:

_____

_____

_____

Spring:

_____

_____

_____

4. Indicate if submitted testimony on student support budget. (Attach copy, if available.)

Council Statement: _____   Letter: _____   Through PTSA: _____   No Testimony: _____

5. Topics discussed during council meetings. (List main topics in order of priority.)

a. _____

b. _____

c. _____

d. _____

e. _____

STUDENT SUPPORT COUNCIL OPERATIONAL PLANS

1. Has the SSAC discussed the student support outcomes for the current year?

   Yes _____   No _____

2. List SSAC activities to help with program implementation and information dissemination.

   _____

   _____

   _____

   _____

   _____

   _____

   _____

   _____

   _____

   _____

   _____

   _____

   _____

3. Describe effectiveness of the student support program in relation to the plan.

Achievements:

_____

_____

_____

_____

_____

_____

_____

_____

4. Problems:

_____

_____

_____

_____

_____

_____

_____

_____

■ WORKSHEET 13.1 (CONTINUED) ■

5. Recommendations:

_____

_____

_____

_____

_____

_____

_____

_____

_____

_____

_____

_____

_____

_____

_____

Has the SSAC reviewed the student support outcomes for the next school year?

Yes _____   No _____

STUDENT SUPPORT ADVISORY COUNCIL REPORT OF ACTIVITIES

1. Describe main SSAC activities and achievements. (Give examples, i.e., helped with scheduling/registration, volunteered in student support office, etc.):

_____

_____

_____

_____

_____

_____

_____

2. Describe any problems encountered. (Give examples, i.e., membership, attendance, administrative support, etc.):

_____

_____

_____

_____

_____

_____

_____

3. Comments, recommendations, and commendations:

_____
_____
_____
_____
_____
_____
_____
_____
_____
_____
_____

CHAIRPERSON OR PERSON TO CONTACT FOR NEXT YEAR

Name: _____

Parent _____ Teacher _____ Student _____ Other _____

Address: _____

Business Phone: _____ Home Phone: _____

Please check: Chairperson _____ or Contact Person _____

■ SUMMARY

The student support advisory council can become a very useful and important adjunct to the student support program. When the decision is made to add an advisory group to a student support program, care must be taken in selecting members who will be representative of the many subpopulations within school district boundaries.

The success of a student support advisory council is a function of how well the meetings are planned. Each meeting should have a purpose, agenda, supporting materials, and leadership to keep members on target for the meeting.

The SSAC calendar is meant to pull together the entire program, making it visible and accountable to the stakeholders—that is, parents, staff, administration, and board of education. The advisory council can become a vocal advocate for the program because they have the opportunity to delve into its intentions and strengths and can recognize the limitations caused by lack of resources. It is potentially the program's most powerful advocate.

■ *A Closing Note from the Authors*

Now that you have examined each element of a comprehensive student support program, it is time to look at the whole to see how the parts are interconnected and interdependent. Each element plays an important role in establishing a solid foundation for achieving student results. Only after the elements are developed and purpose and goals are made clear can program evaluation be designed and implemented. For a student support program to be "evaluable" (capable of being evaluated), its mission, philosophy, goals, competencies must be complete, must be integrated into the mission of the district and school, and must be clearly defined. The program audit form is included in the appendices as a tool that can help determine program evaluability by providing criteria for assessing whether each element is complete.

This model deliberately omits curriculum and other processes for implementing the program. In a pure results-based program, the processes are determined by the student support personnel at each site based on population, resources, environment, and other variables. The world is changing at such a consistent and rapid rate that any suggested processes will probably be out of date before a text can be published. The needs, demands, challenges, and trends of each school and each student are in constant flux. The results-based model provides a vehicle by which student support professionals can reach agreement on the desired goals and competencies for all students.

Appendices B, C, and E–H contain additional tools that can be used in developing the basic program elements as well as samples of materials that might prove helpful for implementation. These are hard-copy tools provided for this book, but in many cases technology can be used to simplify, communicate, and store the data collected for student results (electronic portfolios vs. paper), program results, evaluation data, performance evaluation, and other information needed for ongoing improvement of the program. Please remember in developing, implementing and evaluating a program that the primary purpose of collecting, storing, analyzing, and reflecting on data is to improve the program. Without continual updating, changing, rethinking, and reflecting, any program can become stale and in-effective. However, when everyone on the team is working collaboratively toward the same outcome, utilizing their own skills, interests, and expertise to reach the goals, the program will continue to change and grow, ensuring that each student achieves the desired results.

Appendixes

Sample Glossary

The sample glossary is included to provide an example of the types of words and simplicity of definitions that will ensure that all stakeholders clearly understand the ideas, concepts, and terminology of the results-based student support program. A major mistake made by educators is to assume that all are in agreement when in fact each person on the team may have a different perception of what is meant by terms such as cognitive, developmental, comprehensive, etc. An important step in the formation of the program is to identify any and all words that may need definition and get agreement on the definitions included in the glossary.

Glossary

Accountability is continuous self-evaluation. It requires a goal, performance standard, and timeline. Accountability includes recognizing and following through on a commitment.

Adviser is a certified staff member who is committed to becoming involved in the educational, career, personal, and interpersonal development of her or his advisees.

Advisory is a function of guidance in which certified members of the staff help assigned advisees (students) to plan ahead and proceed successfully through graduation.

Benchmarks are the desired results of student support program goals at specific grade or development levels. The data consist of specific competencies or results with identified criteria for success.

Career/Guidance/Student support center is an educational, career, interpersonal, and personal planning facility housing information and professional services designed to enable an individual or groups of students to determine educational, career, or personal goals. Services are all targeted at helping students develop a viable self-concept enhancing their chosen work values.

Co-learning is a strategy for parent involvement that provides activities for student support professionals and parents to learn from each other and with each other. Examples include inviting parents to attend department meetings in-service sessions, professional organization meetings, etc.

Choice is selection from a set of alternative items, processes, and/or activities.

Co-decision making involves parents in decision-making endeavors, e.g., student decisions and department decisions through the advisory council and participation in individual student placement meetings, etc.

Community connection is the mutual collaboration, support, and participation of families, community members, agencies, and school staff to engage in activities at home, in the community, or at school that directly and positively affect children's success in academic achievement and development.

Competency is developed proficiency in knowledge, attitudes, or skills that are observable, that can be transferred from a learning situation to a real-life situation, and that involve the production of a measurable outcome.

Consultation is collaborative problem solving based on mutual trust to generate commitment to a results-based intervention plan that includes a set of strategies for change. Consultation is also a management technique for influencing others to get things done when you do not have or don't want to use authority.

Co-teaching invites parents to become part of teaching students and staff in areas of expertise, such as career rights, college information, etc.

Co-support utilizes strategies for parents and professionals to work together to support student growth. Examples are fundraising efforts for school activities, booster clubs, Thanksgiving baskets for families, community service, etc.

Counseling is the service that provides both group and one-to-one relationships between students and a professionally competent counselor. The counselor assists the student to integrate and apply self-understanding and understanding of the situation so that she or he can make the wisest and most appropriate choice(s), decision(s), and adjustments.

Curriculum alignment is the process of aligning the program's mission, goals, and competencies with other curricula to ensure that duplication of content and competencies will be kept to a minimum.

Decision making is applying skills and pertinent information to a rational process toward reaching a judgment, determination, conclusion, or course of study.

Developmental guidance is that component of all guidance efforts that fosters planned intervention within educational and other human development programs at all points in the life cycle to vigorously stimulate and actively facilitate the total development of individuals in all areas (personal, social, emotional, moral-ethical, cognitive, and aesthetic) and to promote the integration of the several components into an individual life cycle.

Educational domain refers to a set of competencies that center on ensuring that students acquire life-long learning skills such as knowing how to study, locate, and use resources and knowing their learning styles.

Evaluation is the collection and reporting of information useful in decision making on improving a program or activity to get better results.

Goals are the extension of the mission statement and include specific competencies the student is expected to acquire.

Guidance is an umbrella term that encompasses many facets of an organized program to assist students in acquiring the competencies necessary to develop and implement a post–high school educational and career plan.

Management for results is the management system that has its primary concern the utilization of human resources to produce the desired and agreed upon results.

Means, activities, and/or processes refer to how results are achieved; they are the methodology used to reach a preestablished result.

Monitoring is the process of reviewing data to ascertain if a student or group of students is currently demonstrating the desired goal-related competencies.

Personal domain refers to a set of competencies that centers on ensuring that all students acquire competencies in developing and implementing a balance of family life, nourishment, learning, leisure, exercise, interpersonal activities, and contributions to the community.

Student support program is a results-based program designed and implemented by student support personnel, such as school counselors, school psychologists, social workers, school nurses, and attendance personnel.

System is the "sum total of separate parts working independently and interactive to achieve previously specified results" (Kaufman, 1972).

Worldview refers to one's philosophy of life.

Sample Goals and Competencies

This sample format focuses on goals, subgoals, and competencies. The competencies related to each goal and subgoal are listed by grade level, starting with twelfth grade and ending with lower elementary grades (K–2). Each level is meant to build upon the previous level. Competencies are also sorted by knowledge, attitudes, and skills to match the conceptual model of the program. For example, the educational goal identifies studying and test taking as a subgoal. The competencies for studying and test taking are sorted by grade level and by knowledge, attitudes, and skills. Likewise, the second and third subgoals for the educational domain are followed by related competencies.

The personal/social domain of student competencies has been separated in order to delineate specific areas of personal development. This division also allows for the inclusion of all support personnel to become part of the student success program. These support staff include the school nurse, psychologist, social workers, advisors and others with skills in both interpersonal and personal development. Maintaining a healthy, balanced lifestyle is essential to student success in all areas of life.

■ *Guidance Goals and Competencies in Four Domains*

Educational Domain

GOAL: All students in _____ Schools will acquire and demonstrate competencies in developing an educational program that fulfills their individual learning style, goals, and objectives and provides skills in dealing constructively with and contributing to society.

Each student will acquire and demonstrate competencies in the following:

- Studying and test taking
- Utilizing resources, exercising rights and responsibilities, and following rules and regulations
- Problem solving and planning educational programs

Studying and Test Taking

Knowledge	*Attitudes*	*Skills*
12[1] ■ Show ability to prioritize demands/tasks ■ Identify memorizing techniques ■ Discuss how to prepare for different types of tests ■ Interpret the meanings of cue words used in tests ■ Identify how to organize material being tested ■ Acquire knowledge of how to use test results to diagnose weaknesses in studying techniques ■ Describe time management techniques in test taking ■ Identify strongest and weakest academic aptitudes ■ Explain how to reduce stress in self	■ Seek opportunities to broaden and enhance personal knowledge and skills ■ Use time efficiently to complete assigned work ■ Use stress reduction techniques ■ Acknowledge academic aptitudes	■ Demonstrate effective study skills ■ Demonstrate critical listening skills ■ Manage time in test taking ■ Demonstrate effective stress reduction techniques ■ Select school courses that match academic strengths and weaknesses
9 8 ■ Practice time management principles ■ Describe effective techniques for studying ■ Identify memorizing techniques ■ Discuss how to prepare for different types of tests ■ Interpret the meanings of cue words used in tests ■ Identify how to organize material being tested ■ Describe own learning style ■ Identify own academic strengths	■ Accept responsibility for homework ■ Practice time management in test taking	■ Plan and organize for long-term projects ■ Demonstrate critical listening skills

[1] Numbers in this column indicate that competencies are to be demonstrated by the end of this grade level. The appearance of two numbers indicates application to either junior high or middle school. For example, when numbers 9 and 8 appear, competencies are to be demonstrated by the end of grade 9 in junior high school and grade 8 in middle school. When 5 and 6 appear, competencies are to be demonstrated by the end of grade 5 in K through 5 schools and grade 6 in K through 6 schools.

Studying and Test Taking (cont.)

Knowledge	*Attitudes*	*Skills*
6 ▪ Explain appropriate environment for homework 5 ▪ Discuss organization of one's time and energy to get things done ▪ Interpret meanings of cue words used in tests	▪ Complete required work ▪ Work to strengthen academic weaknesses ▪ Use time management skills	▪ Demonstrate ability to organize time for homework ▪ Demonstrate listening skills ▪ Model memorizing techniques
2 ▪ Identify meanings of cue words used in tests		▪ Organize personal property for the purpose of learning ▪ Demonstrate following directions

Resources, Rights, and Regulations

Knowledge	*Attitudes*	*Skills*
12 ▪ Describe all characteristics of one's school environment ▪ Identify own rights and responsibilities ▪ Describe school environment in terms of rooms and location of personnel ▪ Identify school rules and regulations ▪ List graduation requirements ▪ Know available electives ▪ Describe course prerequisites ▪ Describe available extracurricular activities ▪ Identify available courses at the vocational-technical center ▪ List university, 4-year college, and community college entrance requirements ▪ Describe educational opportunities available in the local community	▪ Recognize the importance of going above and beyond minimal requirements in certain situations ▪ Accept tentative solutions/decisions to problems ▪ Follow school rules and regulations ▪ Assume responsibility for own behavior ▪ Engage in one or more school-related extracurricular activities	▪ Enroll in a course of study to further educational goals ▪ Maintain appropriate classroom and school behavior ▪ Use appropriate resources and opportunities to reach educational goals

Resources, Rights, and Regulations (cont.)

Knowledge	*Attitudes*	*Skills*
9 8 ■ Know courses available at the vocational-technical center ■ Know graduation requirements ■ Know available elective courses ■ Know course prerequisites ■ Know available extracurricular activities	■ Explore alternatives willingly ■ Follow school rules and regulations	■ Engage in appropriate classroom and school behavior
6 5 ■ Identify the role and location of selected school personnel	■ Consider viewpoints of others willingly ■ Use the Media Center resources	■ Maintain appropriate classroom and school-related behavior
2 ■ Identify the location of the school's resources, e.g., principal, Media Center, etc. ■ Recognize the roles of various school personnel ■ Know the school and classroom rules and regulations	■ Engage in appropriate classroom behavior	■ Maintain appropriate classroom and school-related behavior

Problem Solving and Planning

Knowledge	*Attitudes*	*Skills*
12 ■ Prioritize educational needs ■ Describe the systematic problem-solving elements ■ List the parts of a systematic planning process ■ Demonstrate an awareness of decisions made by students using group and individual activities ■ Describe the brainstorming process ■ Recognize the relationship of personal goals and expectations to short- and long-term consequences of actions	■ Search for alternative solutions to problems ■ Plan effectively ■ Accept consequences of decisions	■ Solve problems systematically ■ Demonstrate use of brainstorming techniques in problem solving ■ Use planning techniques in reaching educational goals ■ Use planning skills to select and implement an educational program with emphasis and electives that are consistent with measured abilities, interests, and short- and long-range educational goals ■ Evaluate current educational program to determine success in meeting personal needs and goals

Problem Solving and Planning (cont.)

Knowledge	*Attitudes*	*Skills*
9 8 ▪ List the elements of systematic problem solving ▪ Demonstrate awareness of specific decisions and the consequences of each of the decisions made by groups and individuals	▪ Search for alternative solutions to problems ▪ Use planning skills in completing expected work	▪ Solve problems systematically ▪ Demonstrate brainstorming techniques ▪ Use planning techniques in completing educational goals
6 5 ▪ Name problem-solving elements of needs, solution requirements, alternative solutions, task analysis, and evaluation	▪ Engage in systematic problem solving ▪ Participate in classroom problem-solving and planning process	▪ Demonstrate brainstorming techniques in problem solving ▪ Assess consequences of each alternative solution to a problem
2 ▪ Describe problem-solving processes	▪ Participate in classroom problem-solving and planning processes	

Career/Occupational Domain

GOAL: All students in _____ Schools will acquire and demonstrate competencies in planning and preparing for a career that relates to their career/occupational goals and objectives and to their assessed aptitudes, attitudes, and interests.

    Each student will acquire and demonstrate competencies in the following:

- Knowledge of personal characteristics
- Knowledge of the world of work
- Career decision making and planning
- Finding and keeping employment

Knowledge of Personal Characteristics

Knowledge	*Attitudes*	*Skills*
12 ▪ Describe career/occupational interests, aptitudes, work values, and talents	▪ Acknowledge contributions of self and others	▪ Develop a profile of personal characteristics based on school work, test results, and extracurricular activities[2] ▪ Select and enroll in required and elected courses that match assessed career-related interests, aptitudes, and talents ▪ Evaluate attitudes and behaviors and their effect on functioning in work situations
9 8 ▪ Identify personal career/occupational interests, aptitudes, and talents ▪ Identify positive attitudes toward work ▪ Recognize that schooling is necessary for future careers ▪ Identify sources for information about self ▪ Recognize that each individual is a consumer, producer, and citizen and, as such, has certain rights and responsibilities ▪ Identify personal work strengths and competencies	▪ Select elective courses that relate to assessed career/occupational interests, aptitudes, and talents ▪ Demonstrate an understanding and appreciation of own skills, interests, and attitudes	▪ Demonstrate assessment and consideration of interests, aptitudes, and talents ▪ Develop an individual career plan or profile that includes high school program selections, tentative career goals, and alternative ways to reach those goals using personal characteristics and career information[2] ▪ Analyze abilities and interests in terms of desired occupational areas
6 5 ▪ Compare personal characteristics with those of others	▪ Complete work on time, neatly, and in its entirely ▪ Work cooperatively with team members to complete tasks ▪ Use competencies in completing tasks ▪ Demonstrate appreciation for contributions of self and others	▪ Relate interests and abilities to specific occupational roles

[2] Guidelines will be developed prior to implementation.

Knowledge of Personal Characteristics (cont.)

Knowledge	*Attitudes*	*Skills*
3 ▪ Describe work-related 2 personal characteristics ▪ Identify attitudes and behaviors that help in performing a task ▪ Identify people who are working together toward a common goal and explain how the work of each person contributes to the achievement of that goal	▪ Demonstrate acceptance of others' interests and abilities	
K ▪ Identify basic economic needs and wants and discuss how these are provided ▪ Identify and discuss reasons why some work activities are personally satisfying		

Knowledge of the World of Work

Knowledge	*Attitudes*	*Skills*
12 ▪ Demonstrate knowledge of the nature, structure,[2] and requirements of work ▪ Describe the basic requirements for employment in specific jobs (e.g., special tools, clothing)[2] ▪ Identify and describe various ways of entering the world of work (e.g., vocational training, apprenticeship, cooperative education)[2] ▪ Identify the skills, knowledge, and training required for major occupational categories ▪ Identify criteria for selecting programs, schools, and courses designed to prepare an individual for a job ▪ Identify educational opportunities available in selected careers ▪ Identify occupations that relate to personal interests, aptitudes, and values		▪ Utilize school and community resources to obtain career information

Knowledge of the World of Work (cont.)

Knowledge	*Attitudes*	*Skills*
9 **8** ■ Demonstrate a knowledge of the world of work through occupational categories or career clusters and the associated jobs and requirements ■ Describe three career clusters ■ List five jobs in each of the three clusters ■ List the knowledge, training, and skill requirements in each of the five jobs in the three clusters[2] ■ Identify school subjects that help develop skills, knowledge, and training needed in specific jobs[2] ■ Identify job characteristics that may affect career choice (schedule, benefits, conditions) ■ Recognize that several types of individuals may perform in the same job or occupation ■ Recognize that a range exists of the abilities, interests, and personality traits required for a given job or occupation		■ Use occupational information-seeking skills to match occupational/career requirements with worker traits ■ Classify workers into occupational areas and characterize them as producing goods or services ■ Analyze various work activities in terms of the processes, skills, and concepts derived from basic education necessary to their accomplishment
6 **5** ■ Demonstrate knowledge of broad categories of work and workers (e.g., health workers, food producers, community workers, salespersons) ■ List the advantages that people derive from their work ■ Identify 10 career clusters and list three different jobs in each ■ Develop an awareness of behavior that is appropriate for a particular work situation		■ Classify workers into occupational areas and characterize them as producing goods or services

Knowledge of the World of Work (cont.)

Knowledge	*Attitudes*	*Skills*
2		

Knowledge

2
- Describe the work done by various kinds of people in the community (e.g., mail carrier, sanitation worker, nurse)
- Identify the different kinds of work people do in the home, school, and community
- Identify the skills, tools, and materials needed to perform a job

Career Decision Making and Planning

Knowledge

12
- Examine plans and choices to be made to use available resources effectively, both as consumers and as producers
- Identify employers and job opportunities in the local and surrounding communities
- Match local occupational opportunities with personal interests and abilities
- Identify job characteristics that may affect career choice (e.g., benefits, working conditions), including nontraditional occupations
- Identify occupations that relate to personal interests, aptitudes, and values[2]
- Demonstrate the ability to evaluate programs designed to prepare an individual for a particular job (e.g., private trade school, apprenticeship)
- Develop a profile of personal characteristics based on school work, test results, and extracurricular activities[2]

Attitudes

- Participate in a realistic work situation as part of the school program or as a worker in the community

Skills

- Select educational and training programs in terms of needs, interests, abilities, and values that will assist in converting vocational preference into reality
- Demonstrate the ability to identify and relate personal qualities to employment
- Demonstrate career planning and development skills
- Demonstrate the ability to perform and to learn satisfactorily in a work setting
- Project a career plan that will reflect abilities and interests

Career Decision Making and Planning (cont.)

Knowledge	*Attitudes*	*Skills*
■ Identify alternative personal career goals[2] ■ Identify alternative ways for reaching career goals (immediate and long-range)[2] ■ Demonstrate skills in using school and community resources to obtain career information ■ Develop long-range career goals (3–5 years) as part of the career plan		

	Knowledge	*Attitudes*	*Skills*
9 8	■ Identify the major elements of a career plan ■ Recognize that one's goals and the methods of attaining those goals may change ■ Recognize that career decisions begin early and continue throughout one's lifetime ■ Recognize the importance of alternatives in any plan ■ List sequentially the steps and procedures involved in making education and career decisions[2] ■ List four kinds of information needed to make career decisions ■ Identify three community or school sources of career information[2]	■ Explore a wide range of careers as they reflect interest and abilities ■ Use planning and decision-making competencies in reaching personal goals	■ Make tentative occupational choices in terms of interests, capacities, and values ■ Demonstrate decision-making skills ■ Develop an individual career plan or profile that includes high school program selections, tentative career goals, and alternative ways to reach those goals[2]

Career Decision Making and Planning (cont.)

Knowledge	*Attitudes*	*Skills*
6 5		
■ Describe elements of decision making	■ Use information-seeking skills in making decisions	■ Use planning skills in goal attainment activities
■ Describe elements of planning	■ Finish steps/tasks of plan on time	■ Locate and use information needed in career decision making
■ Identify kinds of information needed in career decision making		
2		
■ Describe elements in making a decision	■ Use decision-making elements in classroom activities	■ Plan classroom-related projects

Finding and Keeping Employment

Knowledge	*Attitudes*	*Skills*
12		
■ Identify qualities and skills that employers commonly seek in job applicants[2]	■ Be punctual with work assignments	■ Demonstrate accurate resume completion
■ Identify educational opportunities available in selected careers[2]	■ Use Career Resource Center materials in job finding and job keeping	■ Demonstrate competence in correctly completing a work application
■ Describe the importance of time in a work setting[2]	■ Cooperate with others in completing tasks	■ Demonstrate skills, attitudes, and behaviors important for a job interview[2]
■ Describe the necessity for correct appearance, punctuality, and task completion	■ Dress appropriately	■ Demonstrate the ability to apply basic skills in a work setting
■ List the major elements in locating work	■ Follow rules and directions	■ Demonstrate basic entry-level skills related to finding and keeping employment
■ Describe the competencies needed to apply for work		■ Demonstrate responsible behavior appropriate for a particular work setting[2]
■ Describe the competencies needed to keep a job		

Finding and Keeping Employment (cont.)

Knowledge	*Attitudes*	*Skills*
9 8 ■ Identify qualities and skills that employers often seek in job applicants ■ Identify potential work opportunities in neighborhood	■ Demonstrate willingness to accept responsibility for one's actions ■ Follow rules and directions	■ Analyze an occupation for desired worker traits ■ Identify and practice attitudes and behaviors that generally apply to any work situation ■ Demonstrate ability to plan work, carry out the plan, and evaluate the effectiveness of the plan ■ Demonstrate interpersonal and human relations skills necessary for successful employment
6 5 ■ Describe worker traits	■ Follow rules and directions ■ Complete work ■ Work as a team member	■ Follow rules and directions
2 ■ Name good worker traits	■ Demonstrate personal pride in work accomplished ■ Demonstrate punctuality and good attendance	■ Demonstrate basic work habits and skills (i.e., interpersonal relationship skills, punctuality) ■ Demonstrate ability to respond positively to direction and instruction ■ Demonstrate ability to relate to peers and teachers ■ Follow classroom rules

Social Domain

GOAL: All students in _____ Schools will acquire and demonstrate competencies in effective interpersonal communication and in recognition of the contributions by self and others.

Each student will acquire and demonstrate competencies in the following:

■ Effective interpersonal communication

■ Recognizing own and others' contributions

Effective Interpersonal Communication

Knowledge	*Attitudes*	*Skills*
12 ▪ Recognize patterns of nonverbal behaviors ▪ Identify own communication style ▪ Identify the ways in which physical and social environment affects one's attitudes toward self, others, and ways of living ▪ Identify persons and organizations from whom one can get assistance with personal concerns	▪ Appreciate unique differences of self and others ▪ Respect each individual's worth and dignity ▪ Recognize feelings of others	▪ Use alternative behaviors in dealing with own needs and feelings ▪ Use skills needed to manage interpersonal relationships ▪ Demonstrate skills for resolving interpersonal conflict ▪ Use styles of interaction that contribute to individual and group goals ▪ Use communication style in contributing to others
9 ▪ Identify personal and interpersonal communication style ▪ Recognize the patterns of one's beliefs and the behavior patterns associated with them[2] ▪ Recognize the effect of one's behavior on others	▪ Contribute to one or more school-related groups ▪ Recognize feelings of others	▪ Demonstrate appropriate communication skills in interpersonal relationships ▪ Demonstrate effective listening skills
6 ▪ Recognize individual capabilities and limitations as related to individual roles ▪ Identify the ways in which physical and social environment affects one's attitudes toward self, others, and ways of living	▪ Recognize feelings of others ▪ Belong to a school-related social group ▪ Recognize that others see one differently from how one perceives self	▪ Demonstrate listening skills ▪ Model specific communication styles ▪ Use *appropriate* coping responses during times of personal stress
3 ▪ Identify communication patterns of self and others ▪ Describe requirements for getting along with others	▪ Recognize feelings of others ▪ Recognize that others may be trusted ▪ Demonstrate a respect for one's environment and the property of others ▪ Cooperate in work and play	▪ Use appropriate styles of communication with classmates

Recognizing Own and Others' Contributions

	Knowledge	Attitudes	Skills
12	■ Identify one's need to belong to a group ■ Identify ways to capitalize on personal strengths ■ Prioritize own needs ■ Identify needs of various societal groups		■ Use social behaviors that show responsibility and independence ■ Use communication style and personality type in contributing to others
9	■ Identify one's need to belong to a group ■ Identify own personal strengths	■ Search for alternatives in fulfilling personal needs ■ Contribute to one or more school-related groups	■ Use social behaviors that show responsibility and independence
6	■ Describe one's need to belong to a group ■ Identify various alternatives for contributing to other students	■ Show respect for others as individuals of worth and dignity	■ Follow rules, accept direction, and take responsibility
3	■ Identify various alternatives for contributing to other students	■ Indicate a wholesome attitude toward self	■ Follow rules, accept direction, and take responsibility

Personal Domain

GOAL: All students in _____ Schools will acquire and demonstrate knowledge, attitudes, and skills in developing personal competencies in leading a healthy, balanced lifestyle.

Each student will acquire and demonstrate competencies in the following:

■ Forming eating patterns that lead to healthy nutritional balance.
■ Effective program of active physical exercise leading to fitness and vitality.
■ Effective plan for positive use of leisure time and recreational activities.
■ Effective personal hygiene and health practices.
■ Positive contributions to family and community leading to a sense of belonging.

Knowledge	Attitudes	Skills
12 ■ Understands nutritional needs of different developmental levels, food groups and appropriate calorie intake ■ Describes importance of a planned program of physical fitness ■ Understands the role of recreation in maintaining a balanced, healthy lifestyle ■ Knowledge of importance of personal hygiene and habits that maintain good health ■ Understands importance of family and community in leading a healthy, balanced lifestyle	■ Understands and practices good nutritional habits ■ Participates in active physical activities ■ Utilizes time for self relaxation, hobbies and/or other positive pastimes ■ Understands and practices good hygiene ■ Participates in family and community activities on a regular basis	■ Prepares and eats a healthy diet including appropriate level of calorie intake and balanced sources of nutrition ■ Maintains a scheduled program of physical fitness activities ■ Skills in planning and using time for recreation ■ Demonstrates skills in maintaining physical hygiene ■ Demonstrates a sense of belonging to family and community groups by contributing to others
9 ■ Identifies elements of a healthy diet and relationship between diet and lifelong health ■ Identify reasons for a planned program of physical fitness ■ Identifies personal skills gained from positive recreational activities ■ Identifies reasons for personal hygiene in self-development ■ Identifies importance of being a contributing member of family and community	■ Eats a balanced diet of nutritional foods ■ Participates in planned, physical activities ■ Utilizes leisure time for relaxation and recreation ■ Demonstrates good personal hygiene and takes pride in cleanliness ■ Contributes time and talent to family and community activities	■ Knowledge of food groups, vitamins, calories and other nutritional facts ■ Uses physical fitness opportunities for self-maintenance ■ Plans personal time for building personal strengths and developing recreational interests ■ Uses skills to maintain personal hygiene ■ Expresses a sense of belonging to family and community
6 ■ Understands food groups and difference between junk food and healthy foods ■ Understands the importance of physical activity to health ■ Identifies available recreational activities at home, school and in the community ■ Describes personal hygiene habits and importance to self ■ Describes own family and community	■ Limits intake of junk food and balances food intake with exercise ■ Enjoys regular physical activities at school and home ■ Chooses at least one recreational activity and becomes involved ■ Practices good personal hygiene ■ Participates willingly in regular family and community activities	■ Develops a balanced eating plan based on personal preferences, and healthy diet ■ Has a plan for spending appropriate amount of time in active physical activity ■ Schedules time for regular recreational activity of choice ■ Allocates time for personal hygiene practices ■ Plans ways to contribute to family and community activities

Sample Benchmarks

- Benchmarks identify desired student accomplishments at specific grades or developmental levels. Benchmarks can be used as a tool to help teachers, parents, and administrators determine the level of attainment for specific groups of skills related to academic success. These are used to determine deficiencies that should be addressed before moving into the next educational level. Therefore, benchmarks are identified for the following transitional levels: grade 3 (lower to upper elementary), grade 6 (elementary to middle school), grades 7, 8, 9, 10, 11, and 12.

- Also included in this section is a simulation for twelfth grade students as they transition from high school to post–high school plans.

- Examples are included for parent/student/counselor review of standards at each transitional level.

Proposed Standards or Benchmarks

Prepared by Sharon K. Johnson, Ed.D., and C. D. Johnson, Ph.D.

It is important to establish benchmarks or standards in order to maintain a consistent school- or district-wide program. These standards allow for external and internal program monitoring of all students as well as individual students. They also provide agreed-upon directions for all pupil services staff.

The following standards are suggestions offered for discussion purposes only. Upon completion of this exercise, there will be consensus on the expected competencies to be demonstrated at specific grade levels. Please note that consensus means "what everyone can live with" and does not mean that all totally agree with each standard.

Grade 3: Each third grade student will demonstrate:

3.1 Appropriate school behaviors and organizational skills.

Criteria: Has materials, is on time, follows teacher's directions, maintains assignment calendar, completes and turns in homework, maintains materials in desk and/or notebook in an organized manner.

***Assessment Strategies:** Teacher's grade book and/or teacher's observations; counselor, psychologist, social worker, principal, or parent observe classroom and homework records; parent validates by signing appropriate homework and homework calendars.

3.2 Interpersonal skills of listening, solving conflicts, and relating appropriately to friends and classmates.

Criteria: Listens to others without interrupting; communicates and plays without conflict behaviors such as yelling, pushing, or name calling; has two or more friends.

Assessment Strategies: Teacher observation and comments; parent validates in parent-counselor conference; pupil service workers observes classroom, playground, and/or small groups.

(Recommend that all information be shared with parents and students in a parent/student/teacher-or-counselor conference.)

Grade 6: Each sixth grade student will demonstrate:

6.1 Appropriate school behaviors and organizational skills.

Criteria: Comes to school with required materials and is on time; follows teacher's directions, rules, and regulations; maintains assignment calendars, completes and turns in homework; organizes and uses notebooks; has established learning ritual at home.

Assessment Strategies: Teacher validates preparation, on time behavior, and

materials; parent validates assignment calendars and rituals; teacher validates if homework assignments are correct/neat, etc.

6.2 Learning strategies that match her/his learning style.

Criteria: Assignments are turned in on time and correct; takes notes on lectures and reading materials; follows directions on teacher-made and standardized tests; describes his/her learning style.

Assessment Strategies: Teacher validates assignment requirements, note taking, and following directions; teacher or counselor validates test-taking skills of following directions, guessing, pacing, being prepared, practice; counselor validates that student knows preferred learning styles and ways to accommodate learning style needs.

6.3 Interpersonal skills in listening, solving conflicts, recognizing contributions of others, and maintaining positive self-esteem.

Criteria: Reflects content and feelings, gives feedback; when in conflict arrives at consensus; describes how others contribute to her/him and the world; and shows a sense of security, identity, belonging, purpose, and personal competence.

Assessment Strategies: Counselor validates in small group counseling or guidance sessions that student can reflect content, reflect feelings, give feedback, and arrive at consensus re: conflict; counselor and parent validate that student has self-knowledge, sense of belonging, purpose, security, and competence.

(Recommend that all information be shared with parents and students in a student-parent-counselor conference.)

Grade 7: Each seventh grade student will demonstrate:

7.1 Appropriate school behaviors and organizational skills.

Criteria: Comes to school with required materials and is on time; follows teacher's

---

*Assessment Strategies may require multiple validations of competencies. Those listed are only examples.

directions, rules, and regulations; maintains assignment calendars, completes and turns in homework; organizes and uses notebooks; has established learning rituals at home; and monitors her/his individual educational progress.

Assessment Strategies: Teacher validates preparation, on-time behavior and materials; parent validates assignment calendars and study rituals; teacher validates if homework assignments meet criteria, e.g., correct/neat, etc.; counselor validates that the subjects-grades-teachers for each grading period are recorded on personal disks, record.

7.2　Learning strategies that match her/his learning style.

Criteria: Assignments are turned in on time and correct; takes notes on lectures and reading materials; follows directions on teacher-made and standardized tests; describes his/her learning style.

Assessment Strategies: Teacher validates assignment requirements, note taking, and following directions; teacher or counselor validates test-taking skills of following directions, guessing, pacing, being prepared, practice; counselor validates that student knows preferred learning style and ways to accommodate learning style needs.

7.3　Skills in preparing a résumé.

Criteria: Knows career interests, learning styles; lists personal skills in learning, working, relating to others, and use of leisure time; lists community contributions; lists membership and awards in organizations such as scouting, churches, junior Red Cross, etc.; hobbies and sports; travel; and awards;

Assessment Strategies: Résumé on file in student's PORTFOLIO that includes evidence of all the above.

7.4　Interpersonal skills in listening, solving conflicts, recognizing contributions of others, and maintaining positive self-esteem.

Criteria: Reflects content and feelings, gives feedback; when in conflict arrives at

consensus; describes how others contribute to her/him and the world; and shows a sense of security, identity, belonging, purpose, and personal competence.

Assessment Strategies: Counselor validates in small group counseling or guidance sessions that student can reflect content, reflect feelings, give feedback, and can arrive at consensus re: conflict; parent and counselor validate that student has self-knowledge, sense of belonging, purpose, security, and competence.

Grade 8: Each eighth grade student will demonstrate:

8.1　Skills in using career information in determining tentative career and educational goals and in résumé updating:

Criteria: Uses career and scholarship resources; completes a four-year educational plan; and completes an update of her/his résumé;

Assessment Strategies: Counselor and parent validates that student's PORTFOLIO contains a copy of an updated résumé and school record; a four-year educational plan approved by parent(s); and each has a copy of the career and scholarship search.

8.2　Skills in interpersonal relationships (listening, cooperatively learning, and appreciating others) and in raising and/or maintaining self-esteem.

Criteria: Reflects content and feelings; provides feedback; uses consensus in solving conflict; shows appreciation of peers and adults, when appropriate; and sets and meets personal goals, has security, belongs to one or more groups;

Assessment Strategies: Counselor or teacher validates that each student has demonstrated the above in small group sessions, classroom activities, or the halls or cafeteria or playground area; parent will validate use of interpersonal skills at home and during leisure time.

Grade 9: Each ninth grade student will demonstrate:

9.1 Knowledge of high school graduation requirements, skills in studying and taking tests, knowledge of school rules and regulations, and skills in educational planning.

Criteria: Enrolled in courses leading to graduation; maintains classroom requirements; at school on time, attends all classes on time, and attends school functions as required; completes a four-year high school plan that meets graduation requirements; shows skills in pacing, following directions, and preparedness in taking tests; and knows learning style preferences.

Assessment Strategies: Counselor and parent(s) validates four-year educational plan as meeting the requirements for graduation; teachers validate following of rules and regulations; teacher and/or counselor validates appropriate test-taking strategies through observation or questions on an exam; and counselors validate student (and parent) knows learning style and how to create a matching learning environment at home.

9.2 Knowledge of work/career strengths, skills in identifying careers that match personal strengths and values, in locating and using career information to determine the requirements to enter a career of choice, in identifying the high school courses to prepare the student to enter the career of choice or to enter an institution of higher learning leading to that career; and knowledge of what is included in a résumé.

Criteria: Lists work skills; uses career search software to identify careers that match work skills and values; identifies high school and post–high school training required to enter a career of choice; and has begun a résumé.

Assessment Strategies: Counselor validates (through reviewing the student's Educational and Career Planning Folder) that student has listed his/her work skills and has offered evidence they are correct; counselor validates that student used career search software to identify one or more careers that match her/his skills and values; and parent, counselor, and/or teacher validates that student has completed a résumé and/or appropriate sections of his/her Educational and Career Planning Folder.

9.3 Skills in listening and solving conflict appropriately, knowledge of contributions of others, and knowledge of his/her style of communication with others.

Criteria: Reflects content and feelings accurately, gives feedback appropriately, and demonstrates arriving at consensus on specific issues or conflicts; describes how everyone gives and is appreciated; and describes his/her personal communication styles based on the Myers-Briggs Temperament Inventory or other personality inventory.

Assessment Strategies: Counselors validate (during small group sessions, viewing video tapes of demonstrations, or classroom activities) that each student has demonstrated she/he can reflect content, feelings, provide feedback, and arrive at consensus as a means of solving conflict; and counselor, teacher, or peer counselor observes and records for each student that she/he has described her/his communication style.

Grade 10: Each 10th grade student will demonstrate:

10.1 Knowledge of courses and extracurricular activities that match her/his academic skills and preparation and social, athletic, or special interests; skills in following school and classroom rules and regulations; skills in preparing for and successfully completing required coursework; and skills in preparing for and taking standardized and teacher-made tests.

Criteria: Is enrolled in and is successfully completing courses required for graduation and selected career preparation; is involved in a minimum of one extracurricular activity; and follows directions, guesses appropriately, and completes all subject-related tests.

Assessment Strategies: Counselor validates that required courses and number of electives are completed satisfactorily; student updates educational progress on computer disk; teacher validates successful test-taking strategies; completes at least one extracurricular activity per semester.

10.2   Skill in updating/preparing personal résumé; attitudes appropriate for successful employment; and knowledge of resources for personal use in career and higher education selection.

   Criteria: Updates résumé on "personal history" disc and provides a copy for the counselor; reports to school, classes, and activities on time in appropriate dress, and participates in ways appropriate for success; demonstrates team membership and commitment; and completes a list of 10 resources—5 in school and 5 out of school—that can be used in deciding on a career and on an institution of higher education, if appropriate.

   Assessment Strategies: Teacher will validate the updated résumé contains work, learning, social, and leisure skills, references, career and educational goals, employment history, community activities, awards, and leisure activities; counselor validates that student has updated records on educational progress, has a minimum of two letters of recommendation.

10.3   Knowledge and skills in building and maintaining self-esteem, handling conflict, selecting and contributing to social groups, and identifying community resources and sources for personal help.

   Criteria: Student describes and shows action that he/she has a sense of security, identity, and belonging; describes her/his purpose and lists personal-social competencies; describes personal problem-solving skills; lists sources of assistance for help with personal problems; and identifies those behaviors of friends that indicate they require assistance.

   Assessment Strategies: A teacher and parent will validate skills and attitudes that show student can increase/maintain self-esteem, including a description of their

(student's) purpose in life and knowledge of their competencies; counselor validates that student has demonstrated adequate skills in solving personal problems; an accurately completed list of resources for help with personal problems will be in the PORTFOLIO; counselor validates student has listed correctly a list of behaviors of others that mandates a referral to a professional helper.

Grade 11: Each eleventh grade student will demonstrate:

11.1   Knowledge of personal academic strengths and deficiencies, college/university/technical school entrance requirements; skills in using career and scholarship search to select institution(s) of higher education and potential financial assistance; and skills in educational planning.

   Criteria: Student records in portfolio her/his academic content strengths (math, language arts, social studies, etc.) and learning strengths (analysis, linear problem solving, creativity, etc.); skills in using computer references in selecting colleges, universities, and sources of financial assistance; and skills in using self-knowledge in completing a post–high school educational plan.

   Assessment Strategies: Counselor validates that student has recorded and student and her/his parents know his/her academic profile of strengths and weaknesses; student has signed up for/or knows/is informed about when to sign up for appropriate test (PSAT, SAT, ACT); teacher or counselor validates student has an updated and accurate résumé and Educational and Career Planning Portfolio.

11.2   Skills in career selection and planning.

   Criteria: Skills in selecting a career that matches assessed interest and abilities; skills in preparing a résumé, job application, and holding a job interview; and skills in planning a career and decision making.

   Assessment Strategies: Counselor and parent validates that student knows his/her career preferences; has the necessary skills and interests to prepare to enter the career; knows how to apply/maintain/advance in/ and leave employment; and has skills in completing a résumé and job application form accurately.

11.3 Skills in relating effectively to others.

Criteria: Skills in reflecting content and feeling, giving feedback to peers and adults, and in solving conflict; and knowledge of how and when to appreciate others' contributions.

Assessment Strategies: Counselor, parent, teacher, and/or peer validates and records that student accurately reflects content and feelings of other students, gives feedback when appropriate, and demonstrates how to arrive at consensus.

(It is HIGHLY RECOMMENDED that each eleventh grade student and her/his parent have an individual career and college planning conference with the counselor. The student's post–high school career and/or college plans should be reviewed and a set of tasks and timelines be specified for the student and agreed upon by the parent. The tasks include use of valid career scholarship information to verify career and educational plans and to identify potential sources of financial assistance. Testing dates, college application dates, and potential college visitations will be planned. The student will update her/ his résumé, secure letters of recommendation, and prepare a sample letter of application.

Grade 12: Each twelfth grade student shall demonstrate:

12.1 Skills in learning.

12.2 Skills in working.

12.3 Skills in developing interpersonal relationships.

Criteria: At a time during spring semester selected by the administration, each (graduating) senior will demonstrate sets of competencies in a series of simulations. The intention of this process is to begin the transition process from high school through a "rites-of-passage" ceremony that will add to the regular graduation activities.

The following is presented for DISCUSSION ONLY and is expected to be modified by local school staff.

12.1 <u>Preparation.</u> Senior girls will be expected to dress in dresses and heels, or they might wear caps and gowns; senior boys with shirts, ties, coats/slacks, and dress shoes. They will appear with their PORTFOLIO and will have been prepared on what to expect.

12.2 <u>Simulation Teams.</u> The teams conducting the competency assessment opportunities will consist of the following: at least one teacher/educator, two parents, and two representatives of the local business/work communities; the team might be chaired by any one member, but it may add more status if the chair is a local business representative or college/university professor.

12.3 The simulations might include the following:

A. Educational planning.

Q1. You selected to attend _____ college/trade schools/ armed forces: Please describe to the committee how you selected the institution, including the factors influencing your decision as well as the decision-making process you followed.

Q2. Colleges/trade schools/armed forces allow for free time to study. What skills do you have and have used that will help you be successful? (Examples: home learning rituals; knowledge and learning/teaching styles; controlling personal stress before, during, and after testing sessions).

B. Career Selection and Planning

C. Job/College Application and Interviewing

D. Interpersonal Problem Solving

E. Leisure

F. "Being a Citizen" Skills and Responsibilities

12.4 During the course of a school day, students will be scheduled to move from station to station. Each team of raters will complete a rating sheet for each student using a predetermined set of criteria.

12.5 A profile will be completed for each student.

An alternative to 12.4 might be for the student to carry from station to station a set of profile sheets (one for each team member) giving one to each rater, who in turn will determine a score, mark it, and sign the sheet . The student then takes it to the next station and follows the same procedures until all simulations are completed.

Examples of Process Expectations or Standards (to Be Considered)

Required parent/student/counselor or teacher individual conference during grades 3, 6, 9, and 11.

- **Grade 3:** Reviews educational progress, home learning rituals, and the establishment of appropriate home learning environment; establishes student's responsibilities for learning. Reinforces communication links between home and school.

- **Grade 6:** Same as grade 3, plus identify specific strengths, review test results including learning styles, review developmental expectations and student responsibilities for learning.

- **Grade 9:** Completes a tentative four-year educational plan. Parent reviews the uses of, and learns how to use, the college, financial aid, and career computer programs. Begins the high school Educational and Career Planning Portfolio. Identifies need for family and school to begin early planning for post–high school educational and career goals through selection of appropriate courses and maintaining rigorous academic expectations.

- **Grade 11:** Career and/or college planning conferences including college applications. Reviews career plans and establishes schedules for tasks to be completed by students and by their parents prior to graduation.

- **Grade 12:** Is encouraged to observe their student's demonstration of competencies.

Sample Needs Assessment

The Individual Guidance Assessment for Educational and Career Planning is a self-reporting instrument for students to assess their aptitudes, academic interests, career interests, and career goals. For counselors the results can be used to identify areas where students want help or feel a deficit. It is recommended that results be given to the students and sent home to parents and a copy retained in the guidance office as a needs assessment when meeting with individuals or groups of students for planning purposes. Large numbers of students requesting help in a specific area provides impetus for the development of guidance curriculum, classroom units, or other delivery systems to address the identified need.

Educational and Career Planning Individual Guidance Assessment Middle/Junior High School—Form B

Developed by C. D. Johnson, Ph.D.
Sharon K. Johnson, Ed.D.

DIRECTIONS:

The INDIVIDUAL GUIDANCE ASSESSMENT is an opportunity for you to assess your aptitudes, academic interests, career interests, and career goals.

This is <u>NOT</u> a test. There are no right or wrong answers.
This is a <u>self-reporting inventory</u>. The items pertain to your potential educational plans and career choices. Some items are designed so that you may indicate areas where you would like or need assistance. For example, one item allows you to indicate a need for help in test-taking skills while another item allows you to indicate a need for help in finding a job.

The results (1) will be used by the counselors to assist you in areas of your identified needs and (2) will be mailed home to your parent(s). There will be no permanent record of your responses retained by the school. You will be given a copy of your PROFILE to use in planning your educational and career goals.
There may be words, terms, or comments on the IGA that you do not understand. <u>You are encouraged to ask for information or explanation</u>.

REMEMBER: THIS IS NOT A TEST. THIS IS AN OPPORTUNITY FOR YOU TO ASSESS YOUR EDUCATIONAL AND CAREER PLANNING GUIDANCE NEEDS.

USE A PENCIL ONLY.

1. In planning my school program, I need the most help in knowing about: (From the following list, select only <u>ONE</u> or <u>TWO</u>—no more than two—areas in which you would like help.)
   A. Graduation requirements.
   B. Possible elective or alternative courses.
   C. Course prerequisites (aptitudes, abilities, and skills).
   D. Career possibilities of elective courses.
   E. Extracurricular activities (sports, clubs, student activities).
   F. My rights and responsibilities as a student.
   G. Knowing what courses are available for me at the Vocational-Technical Center.
   H. No help needed at this time.
   I. All the above.

2. I do my best work in: (Select <u>ONE</u> or <u>TWO</u> areas in which you do your best work.)
   - A. Giving oral reports in front of the class.
   - B. Making drawings and designs (art work).
   - C. Doing arithmetic problems.
   - D. Writing compositions.
   - E. Discussing topics in social studies.
   - F. Doing science experiments.
   - G. Making things with my hands.
   - H. Taking part in physical education.
   - I. Helping at home.
   - J. I am not sure what I do best.

3. I need the most help to improve my schoolwork in: (Select <u>ONE</u>, <u>TWO</u>, or <u>THREE</u> areas in which you need the most help.)
   - A. Giving oral reports in front of the class.
   - B. Making drawings and designs (art work).
   - C. Doing arithmetic problems.
   - D. Writing compositions.
   - E. Discussing topics in social studies.
   - F. Doing science experiments.
   - G. Making things with my hands.
   - H. Taking part in physical education.
   - I. I am not sure what I need the most help with.
   - J. I do not need help at this time.

4. I estimate my grades since 5/6th grades to be:
   - A. Mostly As.
   - B. Mostly As and Bs.
   - C. Mostly Bs.
   - D. Mostly Bs and Cs.
   - E. Mostly Cs.
   - F. Mostly Cs and Ds.
   - G. Mostly Ds.
   - H. Mostly Ds and Fs.

5. Compared with my ability, I think my grades are:
   - A. Considerably below my ability.
   - B. A little below my ability.
   - C. About right for my ability.
   - D. Higher than I expected.
   - E. I don't know my abilities.

6. My favorite hobby is:
   - A. Playing and/or watching sports.
   - B. Building models, art work, or crafts.
   - C. Singing or playing musical instruments.
   - D. Sewing and cooking.
   - E. Fishing and hunting or working in the garden or yard.
   - F. Raising pets.
   - G. Collecting things.
   - H. Fixing and repairing things.
   - I. Reading.
   - J. I am not sure what my favorite hobby is.

7. I like the following school subject best: (Select <u>ONE</u> or <u>TWO</u> subjects you like best.)
   - A. English.
   - B. Foreign Language.
   - C. Mathematics.
   - D. Social Studies.
   - E. Science.
   - F. Fine Arts, Music
   - G. Home Economics.
   - H. Industrial Arts.
   - I. Physical Education.
   - J. I am not sure which school subject I like best.

8. To be more successful in school, I need help in: (Select <u>ONE</u> or <u>TWO</u> areas in which you need help.)
   - A. Knowing how to study better.
   - B. Knowing how to get organized.
   - C. Knowing how I learn best.
   - D. Knowing how to do better in tests.
   - E. Knowing how to take class notes better.
   - F. All the above.
   - G. I do not need help at this time.

9. I like to spend my leisure time in: (Select <u>ONE</u> or <u>TWO</u> of the following.)
   - A. Reading.
   - B. Watching TV.
   - C. Listening to the radio.
   - D. Being with friends and going to parties.
   - E. Making things (building, sewing, cooking, models, etc.).
   - F. Going to shows.
   - G. My hobbies (collecting stamps, coins, etc.).
   - H. Playing and/or watching sports on weekends and after school.
   - I. Clubs (Scouts, Y-Clubs, etc.).
   - J. I am not sure how I would like to spend most of my leisure time.

10. I would like to know how I compare with others my age in: (Select <u>ONE</u> or <u>TWO</u> areas about which you would like to know.)
    - A. School achievement.
    - B. Things I like to do.
    - C. Things I want or things I think are important.
    - D. How I look.
    - E. Getting along with others.

F. Getting along with me.

G. What hobbies I have.

H. None of the above.

I. All the above.

J. I am not sure what I would like most to know.

11. I would like to know more about me in regard to:

A. What can help me in school to get better grades.

B. What can help me have more fun.

C. What can help me earn more money now.

D. What can help me choose a career.

E. What can help me have more friends.

F. Other.

G. I do not need help at this time to know more about me.

12. At this time, I am most interested in: (Select ONE, TWO, or THREE areas of interest.)

A. Outdoor work.

B. Mechanical work.

C. Working with numbers.

D. Scientific work.

E. Working with my hands.

F. Sales work, advertising, public relations.

G. Work that uses my artistic ability.

H. Work that involves reading and writing.

I. Work that uses my musical ability.

J. Work in which I am of direct service to other people.

13. In planning my career (life's work) for the future, at this time, I need the most help in:

A. What career fields are there (kinds of jobs available).

B. What education is required for certain jobs.

C. What do people do in different jobs (e.g., doctor, store manager, truck driver, etc.).

D. Learning how much a job pays.

E. Where jobs are found.

F. What are different ways of getting certain jobs.

G. Which jobs may or may not be needed in the future.

H. All the above.

I. I do not need help at this time in planning my career.

J. Other.

14. I need more information about how my future career (or job) might have something to do with: (Select ONE or TWO of the following.)

A. The way I live.

B. Where I might live.

C. The use of my free time (recreation).

D. My health and physical condition.

E. My choice of friends and associates.

F. My dress and how I wear my hair.

G. All the above.

H. I do not need more information at this time.

I. Other.

15. In terms of planning for my future career, at this time, I am most interested in information about: (Select ONE or TWO areas of interest.)

A. Jobs that require a high school diploma and special training.

B. Jobs where you receive training on the job.

C. Jobs that require special apprenticeship training.

D. Jobs that require one or two years of college.

E. Jobs that require four years or more of college.

F. I am not interested in career information at this time.

G. I am not sure what type of information I have the most interest in at this time.

H. All the above.

16. I think it will be most important in the future for me to choose:

A. Courses where my abilities are strong and I know I can be successful.

B. Courses where my interest is high and I want to know more about the subject.

C. Courses that are important to my future educational and career plans.

D. All the above.

E. I am not sure what will be most important for me.

F. Other.

17. My biggest problem at this time in deciding on what courses to take in the future will be that: (Select ONE or TWO of the following.)

A. I don't know whether I am really interested in certain courses.

B. I don't know whether I can do the work required in certain courses.

C. I don't know what some courses are all about.

D. I don't know whether certain courses will help me with my future job or career.

E. All the above.

F. I am not sure at this time what my biggest problem will be in deciding.

G. Other.

18. I am exploring career and job opportunities at this time by: (Select <u>ONE</u> or <u>TWO</u> of the following.)

A. Attending educational programs outside of school (science fairs, musical programs, auto shows, traveling, etc.).

B. Engaging in part-time work (delivering papers, baby sitting, gardening, etc.).

C. Participating in education outside of regular school (summer school, courses at church, scouting, private lessons in music, art, language, dancing, etc.).

D. Enrolling in exploratory career courses (science, shop, art, foreign language, etc.).

E. Talking it over with someone (parents, teachers, or counselors).

F. Does not apply (no tentative career plans at this time).

G. I have no progress to date in exploring career and job opportunities.

H. Participating in one of the programs at the Vocational-Technical Centers.

19. I would like additional help in learning: (Select <u>ONE</u> or <u>TWO</u> of the following.)

A. What kinds of jobs are available to students my age.

B. How much part-time jobs pay.

C. Where I can look for part-time and summer jobs.

D. How do I make out an application form.

E. What is the proper way to interview for a job.

F. How do I get a social security card.

G. Where do I get a work permit.

H. All the above.

I. I need no help at this time.

J. Other.

20. I would like some assistance in my school courses at this time in: (Select <u>ONE</u> or <u>TWO</u> of the following.)

A. How to study better.

B. How to complete assignments.

C. How to earn satisfactory grades.

D. How to maintain satisfactory classroom behavior.

E. How to use my time better.

F. All the above.

G. I do not need help at this time in my school courses.

21. I have a physical handicap that might limit my educational and career plans:

A. Yes.

B. No.

C. I am not certain whether I have a physical handicap that will limit my educational and career plans.

22. Which of the statements listed below describes me best at this time: (Select <u>ONE</u>, <u>TWO</u>, or <u>THREE</u> of the following.)

A. I can describe my interests clearly.

B. I have a good idea of what my test scores indicate.

C. I can explain how the courses I am taking will fit into my future plans.

D. I know what courses are hard for me to do.

E. I have some idea of how much training is required for different jobs.

F. I know the things that I can do easily and well.

G. All the above.

H. I am not sure which of the statements describes me best at this time.

23. Which of the statements listed below describes me least at this time: (Select <u>ONE</u>, <u>TWO</u>, or <u>THREE</u> of the following.)

A. I can describe my interests clearly.

B. I have a good idea of what my school test scores indicate.

C. I can explain how the courses I am taking will fit into my future plans.

D. I know what courses are hard for me to do.

E. I have some idea of how much training is required for different jobs.

F. I know the things that I can do easily and well.

G. All the above.

H. I am not sure which statement is least like me at the present time.

Educational and Career Planning Individual Guidance Assessment High School—Form C

Developed by Clarence D. Johnson, Ph.D., and Sharon K. Johnson, Ed.D.

DIRECTIONS:

The INDIVIDUAL GUIDANCE ASSESSMENT is an opportunity for you to assess your skills, academic interests, career interests, and career goals.

This is <u>NOT</u> a test. There are no right or wrong answers.

This is a <u>self-reporting inventory</u>. The items pertain to your potential educational plans and career choices. Some items are designed so that you may indicate areas where you would like or need assistance. For example, one item allows you to indicate a need for help in test-taking skills while another item allows you to indicate a need for help in finding a job.

The results (1) will be used by the counselors to assist you in areas of your identified needs and (2) will be mailed home to your parent(s). There will be no permanent record of your responses retained by the school. You will be given a copy of your PROFILE to use in planning your educational and career goals.

There may be words, terms, or comments on the IGA that you do not understand. <u>You are encouraged to ask for information or explanation</u>.

REMEMBER: THIS IS NOT A TEST. THIS IS AN OPPORTUNITY FOR YOU TO ASSESS YOUR EDUCATIONAL AND CAREER PLANNING GUIDANCE NEEDS.

USE A PENCIL ONLY.

1. In planning my school program, I need the most help in knowing about: (From the following list, select only <u>ONE</u>.)
    A. Graduation requirements.
    B. Possible elective or alternative courses.
    C. Course prerequisites (aptitudes, abilities, and skills).
    D. Extracurricular activities (sports, clubs, student activities).
    E. None of the above.

2. In planning my school program, I need the most help in knowing about: (From the following list, select only <u>ONE</u>.)
    A. Extracurricular activities (sports, clubs, student activities).
    B. My rights and responsibilities as a student.
    C. Knowing what courses are available for me at the Vocational-Technical Center.
    D. No help needed at this time.
    E. All the above.

3. I do good work in: (Select <u>ONE</u>.)
    A. Giving oral reports in front of the class.
    B. Making drawings and designs (art work).
    C. Doing arithmetic problems.
    D. Writing compositions.
    E. None of the above.

4. I do good work in: (Select <u>ONE</u>.)
    A. Discussing topics in social studies.
    B. Doing science experiments.
    C. Making things with my hands.
    D. Taking part in physical education.
    E. I am not sure what I do best.

5. I need help to improve my schoolwork in:
    (Select <u>ONE</u>.)
    A. Giving oral reports in front of the class.
    B. Making drawings and designs (art work).
    C. Doing arithmetic problems.
    D. Writing compositions.

6. I am not sure what I need the most help
    with: (Select <u>ONE</u>.)
    A. Discussing topics in social studies.
    B. Doing science experiments.
    C. Making things with my hands.
    D. Taking part in physical education.
    E. I do not need help at this time.

7. I estimate my grades since 5/6 grades to be:
    A. Mostly As and some Bs.
    B. Mostly Bs with some As and Cs.
    C. Mostly Cs with some Bs, As.
    D. Mostly Cs and Ds.
    E. Mostly Ds and Fs.

8. Compared with my ability, I think my
    grades are:
    A. Considerably below my ability.
    B. A little below my ability.
    C. About right for my ability.
    D. Higher than I expected.
    E. I don't know what my abilities are.

9. My favorite hobby is:
    A. Playing and/or watching sports.
    B. Building models, art work, or crafts.
    C. Singing or playing musical instruments.
    D. Sewing and cooking.
    E. None of the above.

10. My favorite hobby is:
    A. Fishing and hunting or working in the
       garden or yard.
    B. Raising pets.
    C. Collecting things.
    D. Reading.
    E. I am not sure what my favorite hobby is.

11. I like the following school subject best:
    (Select <u>ONE</u>.)
    A. English.
    B. Foreign Language.

    C. Math.
    D. Social Studies.

12. I like the following elective subject best:
    (Select ONE.)
    A. Fine Arts, Music.
    B. Home Economics.
    C. Industrial Arts.
    D. Physical Education.
    E. I am not sure which school subject I
       like best.

13. To be successful in school, I need help in:
    (Select only <u>ONE</u>.)
    A. Knowing how to study better and to get
       organized.
    B. Knowing how I learn best.
    C. Knowing how to do better in tests.
    D. Knowing how to take class notes better.
    E. All the above, or I do not need help at
       this time.

14. I like to spend my leisure time in: (Select <u>ONE</u>.)
    A. Reading.
    B. Watching TV.
    C. Listening to the radio.
    D. Being with friends and going to parties.
    E. None of the above.

15. I like to spend my time in: (Select <u>ONE</u>.)
    A. Making things (building, sewing,
       cooking, models, etc.)
    B. Going to shows.
    C. My hobbies (collecting stamps, coins, etc.)
    D. Playing and/or watching sports on
       weekends and after school.
    E. I am not sure how I would like to spend
       most of my leisure time.

16. I would like to know how I compare with
    others my age in: (Select <u>ONE</u>.)
    A. School achievement.
    B. Things I like to do.
    C. Things I want or things I think are
       important.
    D. How I look.

17. I would like to know how I compare with
    others my age in: (Select <u>ONE</u>.)
    A. Getting along with others.
    B. Getting along with me.
    C. What hobbies I have.
    D. None of the above.
    E. I am not sure what I would like most
       to know.

18. I would like to know more about me in regard to:
    A. What can help me in school to get better grades.
    B. What can help me have more fun.
    C. What can help me earn more money or choose a career.
    D. What can help me have more friends.
    E. Other, or I do not need help at this time to know more about me.

19. At this time I am most interested in: (Select ONE.)
    A. Outdoor work.
    B. Mechanical work.
    C. Working with numbers.
    D. Scientific work.
    E. Working with my hands.

20. At this time, I am also interested in: (Select ONE.)
    A. Sales work, advertising, public relations.
    B. Work that uses my artistic ability.
    C. Work that involves reading and writing.
    D. Work that uses my musical ability.
    E. Work in which I am of direct service to other people.

21. In planning my career (life's work) for the future, at this time, I need the most help in:
    A. What career fields are there (kinds of jobs available).
    B. What education is required for certain jobs.
    C. What do people do in different jobs (e.g., doctor, store manager, truck driver, etc.)
    D. Learning how much a job pays.
    E. None of the above.

22. In planning my career (life's work) for the future, at this time, I need the most help in:
    A. Where jobs are found.
    B. What are different ways of getting certain jobs.
    C. Which jobs may or may not be needed in the future.
    D. All the above.
    E. I do not need help at this time in planning my career.

23. I need more information about how my future career (or job) might have something to do with: (Select ONE.)
    A. The way I live.
    B. Where I might live.
    C. The use of my free time (recreation).

    D. My health and physical condition.
    E. None of the above.

24. I would like additional information about how my career (or job) might have something to do with (Select ONE.)
    A. My choice of friends and associates.
    B. My dress and how I wear my hair.
    C. All the above.
    D. I do not need more information at this time.
    E. Other.

25. In terms of planning for my future career, at this time I am most interested in information about: (Select ONE.)
    A. Jobs that require a high school diploma and special training.
    B. Jobs where you receive training on the job.
    C. Jobs that require special apprenticeship training.
    D. Jobs that require one or two years of college.
    E. None of the above.

26. In terms of planning for my future career, I would like information about: (Select ONE.)
    A. Jobs that require four years or more of college.
    B. I am not interested in career information at this time.
    C. I am not sure what type of information I have the most interest in at this time.
    D. All of the above.
    E. Other.

27. I think it will be most important in the future for me to choose:
    A. Courses where my abilities are strong and I know I can be successful.
    B. Courses where my interest is high and I want to know more about the subject.
    C. Courses that are important to my future educational and career plans.
    D. All the above.
    E. I am not sure what will be most important for me.

28. My biggest problem at this time in deciding on what courses to take in the future will be that: (Select ONE.)
    A. I don't know whether I am really interested in certain courses.
    B. I don't know whether I can do the work required in certain courses.

C. I don't know what some courses are all about.

D. I don't know whether certain courses will help me with my future job or career.

E. All the above, or I am not sure at this time what my biggest problem will be in deciding.

29. I am exploring career and job opportunities at this time by: (Select ONE.)

A. Attending educational programs outside of school (science fairs, musical programs, auto shows, traveling, etc.).

B. Engaging in part-time work (delivering papers, babysitting, gardening, etc.).

C. Participating in education outside of regular school (summer school, courses at church, scouting, private lessons in music, art, language, dancing, etc.).

D. Enrolling in exploratory career courses (science, shop, art, foreign language, etc.).

E. Other.

30. I would like additional help in learning: (Select ONE.)

A. What kinds of jobs are available to students my age.

B. How much part-time jobs pay.

C. Where I can look for part-time and summer jobs.

D. How do I make out an application form.

E. None of the above.

31. I would like additional help in learning:

A. What is the proper way to interview for a job.

B. How do I get a social security card.

C. All the above.

D. I need no help at this time.

E. Other.

32. I would like some assistance in my school courses at this time in: (Select ONE or TWO of the following.)

A. How to study better and how to complete assignments.

B. How to earn satisfactory grades.

C. How to maintain satisfactory classroom behavior.

D. How to use my time better.

E. I do not need help at this time in my school courses.

33. I have a physical handicap that might limit my educational and career plans.

A. Yes.

B. No.

C. I am not certain whether I have a physical handicap that will limit my educational and career plans.

34. Which of the statements listed below describes me best at this time: (Select ONE.)

A. I can describe my interests clearly.

B. I have a good idea of what my test scores indicate and the things I do easily and well.

C. I can explain how the courses I am taking will fit into my future plans.

D. I know what courses are hard for me to do.

E. All the above, or I am not sure which of the statements describes me best at this time.

Sample Program Audit Form

The program audit is a tool to determine the evaluability of a results-based student support program. It is a monitoring tool that provides criteria for assessing the level of completeness of each program element. Appropriate use of this tool provides counselors and administrators with data on the consistency and status of the current program efforts. When all the program elements are complete and are being implemented, the program is ready for evaluation.

Audit Criteria for Results-Based School Guidance Programs

Purpose: The purpose of a program audit is to provide administrators and counselors with criteria to use in monitoring the school-based, results-based guidance program to determine a program's evaluability. The program elements and criteria for evaluability are identified for each element. Counselors, administrators, parents, staff, and others are encouraged to participate in the auditing process. A program is considered evaluable (ready for evaluation) once all elements are completed and being implemented.

The following guidance program elements and related criteria are suggested to assist each school and school district in their efforts to develop the results-based guidance program. Each element has a set of criteria for determining the completeness and consistency of each element within the whole program.

The 12 elements of the program are divided into two categories: **Results** and **Means**.

RESULTS: Mission, Philosophy, Conceptual Model, Goals, and
Competencies

MEANS: Management System, Results Agreements, Needs
Assessment, Results Plans, Student Monitoring, Master
Calendar, Advisory Council

Elements and Criteria: A Checklist

The elements and criteria are presented with an auditing system intended to help guide counselors and other student support personnel in developing a complete and consistent results-based guidance program. The following scale can be used to validate the school personnel's efforts in monitoring program progress.

_____ 1. Not Started   When all criteria statements are checked "No."
_____ 2. Working   When one or more criteria are met.
_____ 3. Completed   When all criteria are met.
_____ 4. Implementing   When evidence of implementation is validated.
_____ 5. Not applicable   When program element is not being utilized.

Results

1. Mission of Guidance

The mission articulates the intentions of the guidance program. It is the long-range desired impact, i.e., what is desired for all students five to ten years after graduation.

_____1.1   Written with the student as the primary client.
_____1.2   Written for all students.
_____1.3   Indicates categories of guidance-related content or skills to be learned.
_____1.4   Links with the statement of vision, purpose, or mission of the district and the school.

2. Philosophy

The philosophy is a set of principles that guide the development, implementation, and evaluation of the program.

_____2.1   Addresses all students.
_____2.2   Focuses on primary prevention and student development.
_____2.3   Identifies people to be involved in the delivery of activities.
_____2.4   Identifies who will plan and manage the program.
_____2.5   Defines the management system to be used.
_____2.6   Indicates how the program will be evaluated and by whom.
_____2.7   Indicates who will be responsible for monitoring students' progress.
_____2.8   Indicates when and how counselors will maintain their professional competencies.
_____2.9   Indicates the ethical guidelines for the program.

3. Conceptual Model

A conceptual model of guidance provides a structure for the definition of goals and related competencies and is developmental in nature.

_____3.1   Focuses on all domains of guidance.
_____3.2   Identifies a framework for organization of goals and competencies (knowledge, attitudes and skills).

_____3.3   Identifies the developmental structure for the guidance program from pre-K or K–12 (or beyond).

4. Goals

Goals are the extension of the statement of purpose or mission and provide the desired student results to be achieved by the time the student leaves the school system.

_____4.1   Goals are expressed in terms of what students are expected to achieve.

_____4.2   Goals demonstrate linkage with the guidance mission, the school's mission, and student expected results (ESLRs).

_____4.3   Goals include knowledge, attitudes, and skills in the following domains:
 _____ Learning to learn (educational domain)
 _____ Learning to work (career domain)
 _____ Learning to relate to self and others (personal/social domain)
 _____ Learning to use leisure time effectively (wellness/leisure domain)

5. Competencies

Competencies are knowledge, attitudes, or skills that are observable and can be transferred from a learning situation to a real-life situation and that involve the production of a measurable outcome. Competencies are indicators that a student is making progress toward the guidance goals.

_____5.1   Are directly related to the goal.
_____5.2   Are developmental.
_____5.3   Are measurable.

Means

6. Management System

The management system is the process by which accountability for results is established and indicates who will be responsible for which students acquiring predetermined competencies.

_____6.1   Counselors and administrators agree on assignments of counselors.

_____6.2   Counselors have identified specific results they are accountable for.

_____6.3   All goals are covered.

_____6.4   All students are included in the results.

_____6.5   There is a clear division between assumed accountability for results and assigned duties.

_____6.6   There is an established timeline for reporting evidence of results attained.

_____6.7   There are a means and process in place to monitor all students' guidance progress.

7. Results Agreements

Results agreements are statements of responsibility by each counselor specifying the results and students the counselor is accountable for. These agreements are negotiated with and approved by the designated administrator.

____7.1   The results domain is clearly delineated.
____7.2   Results are stated in terms of what will be demonstrated by the student, parent, and staff member so the results can be documented.
____7.3   The results agreement is consistent with program goals and competencies.
____7.4   The administrator responsible for the guidance program has been actively involved in the negotiation of the results agreement.
____7.5   There is a results agreement addressing every aspect of the program, educational/academic, career, personal/social, and leisure activities.

8. Needs Assessment

Needs are identified discrepancies between the desired results and the results currently being achieved.

____8.1   The assessed needs are related to the guidance goals and competencies.
____8.2   The guidance needs are student-based discrepancies.

9. Results Plans

For every competency or result assumed by counselors, there must be a plan for how the responsible counselor intends to achieve the desired competency or result. Each plan contains (1) desired result, (2) where and how competencies will be achieved, (3) who is responsible for delivery of competency, (4) time to be completed, (5) materials required, (6) criteria for success, and (7) means of evaluation. A results plan is completed by each counselor.

____9.1   Written plans are on file with the administrator in charge of guidance.
____9.2   Plans include specific competency(ies), who/when/where program will be done, what activities will be used, who is accountable for completion of the plan, specified completion date, materials required, criteria of success, and means of evaluation or data collection.
____9.3   Plans have been reviewed and signed by the principal.

10. Monitoring Students' Progress

Monitoring students' guidance progress is the process of ensuring that each student acquires the identified competencies. The process includes a responsible adult in the student's life (counselor, teacher, parent, administrator, other) observing competency demonstration, and recording the verification on a form (Planning Folder, Portfolio, mark-sense form, computer disk, or other documentation).

____10.1   Counselors are accountable for all students.

____10.2   There is an established means to monitor students' progress in guidance-related competencies, including academic achievement.

____10.3   Each student has a means to document own progress, knows where documentation is kept, and how to access documentation.

____10.4   Monitoring activities are delineated by grade level.

11. Master Calendar

A master calendar of guidance events is developed and published to encourage students, parents, teachers, and administrators to know what is scheduled; when and where activities will be held; and to plan ahead to ensure active participation in the program.

____11.1   A master calendar exists.

____11.2   The master calendar identifies grade level(s), date, and activity.

____11.3   Master calendar is published and distributed to appropriate persons: students, staff, parents, and community.

12. Advisory Council

An advisory council is a group of persons appointed to audit the guidance goals and competencies and to make recommendations to the department, principal, and/or the superintendent. The membership has representation of groups effected by the guidance program: students, parents, teachers, counselors, administrators, and community members.

____12.1   An Advisory Council has been organized and has established meeting dates and has identified tasks.

____12.2   The Advisory Council has appropriate representative membership.

____12.3   Recommendations and reports are submitted to appropriate persons in a timely manner.

Program Evaluation

The primary purpose of program evaluation is to provide evidence of guidance program success. Student competency evaluation provides counselors a means to identify where to focus their efforts to improve one or more aspects of the program. Evaluation can also be used to show that a specific goal has or has not been reached. The primary purpose for collecting information is to guide future actions to improve future results. "The purpose of evaluation is . . . to improve Stufflebeam, D., et al. (1971)" (Stufflebeam, Foley, Gephart, Guba, Hammond, Merriman, and Provus, 1971).

- **Competency evaluation:** This assessment of student progress is done by the counselor, teacher, or other staff member immediately after a process is completed. The specific knowledge, attitudes, and skills demonstrated by a student at a specific time is measured.

- **Goal evaluation:** This evaluation is done when the student is ready to graduate from the school or program. It measures the cumulative achievement by students of guidance-related competencies.

- **Mission evaluation:** This evaluation measures the long-term societal consequences of the guidance program. The intentionality of the program is measured 3–5–10 years after the student leaves the institution.

- **Impact evaluation:** Impact results are those that occur as a consequence of a planned, implemented, and evaluated results-based program. For example, the intended impact of ensuring that all students learn test-taking skills is the attainment of higher test scores. However, impact results usually involve a number of variables only some of which are ascribed to the guidance program. School profile data is used to determine impact.

- **Benchmark evaluation:** Some programs define specific times in a student's education when an assessment of progress toward guidance results is helpful in planning for the next phase of education. Frequently these points occur when a child moves from primary to upper elementary (grade 3 or 4), when the student moves into middle/intermediate or junior high school, when the student moves to high school, and in eleventh grade, one year before graduation to allow time for remediation of competencies not yet attained. Benchmark evaluation also provides data for counselors to make mid-course corrections if several students are not at the expected level of achievement.

____1. Competencies are evaluated and reported.
____2. Goal evaluation is completed and reported.
____3. Follow-up data collection system is implemented and findings reported.
____4. Evaluation data is analyzed and the findings are used to improve the program.

Sample Educational and Career Planning Portfolio

The Educational and Career Planning Portfolio provides a visual path for students and parents to understand the process, information, and experiences that will prepare students for future success. The portfolio can begin as early as upper elementary and middle school but is most crucial as a tool for high school students. The contents of the portfolio record the progress students have made in developing competencies and plans for their educational and career futures. Parents and students are encouraged to add to and review the portfolio on a regular basis. In addition to educational records, other family and community activities should be regularly documented and added to the portfolio to provide a comprehensive view of the student's interests, accomplishments, talents, and contributions.

■ *Student Educational and Career Planning Portfolio*

Student Name _____

Address _____

Telelephone Number _____

Birthdate _____

Graduation Date _____

School _____

Principal _____

Counselor _____

■ *Personal Information*

The personal information section is to be filled in by you. The content is information that is frequently requested on applications, and various other forms. If you do not know, or are unaware of your strengths, ask your parents, friends, counselors, teachers, or administrators, or leave it blank. If you have any questions or concerns, please see your counselor or administrator, at your earliest convenience.

Full Name _____   Date of Birth _____ / _____ / _____

Social Security _____ - _____ - _____   Driver's License (State) _____

Place of Birth _____   Passport No. _____

Family Address _____

Father's Name _____

Mother's Name _____

Schools Attended:

Grade	Name	Address		Teacher and/or Principal
K				
1				
2				
3				
4				
5				
6				
7				
8				
9				
10				
11				
12				

Honors/Awards (Please identify honor/award by age or grade, and place)

Title of Honor/Award   Age/Grade   Where

_____

_____

_____

_____

(Example: Perfect Attendance, Honor Roll, Scouting Merit Badges, Church Awards)

■ *Competencies*

School: My best performance has been in the following subjects:

____ English	____ U.S. History	____ Calculus	____ Physics
____ Literature	____ Economics	____ Computers	____ Sports
____ Speech	____ Current Affairs	____ Mechanics	____ Spanish
____ Drama	____ Physical Education	____ Music	____ French
____ U.S. Gov't.	____ Journalism	____ General Science	____ German
____ Art	____ Carpentry	____ Life Science	____ Russian
____ Home Econ.	____ General Math	____ Physical Science	____ Latin
____ Drafting	____ Algebra 1	____ Physiology	____ Other
____ Geography	____ Algebra 2	____ Biology	____ _____
____ World History	____ Geometry/Trigonometry	____ Chemistry	____ _____

■ **Skills:** My best skills are:

(Example: Writing, algebra, speaking, taking tests, doing homework, studying)

_____   _____

_____   _____

_____   _____

_____   _____

■ **Social Skills:** My best social skills are:

(Ex: listening, handling conflict, handling stress, meeting new people, making friends)

_____   _____

_____   _____

_____   _____

_____   _____

(You are encouraged to ask your friends, parents, counselors, and teachers what they perceive as your personal/social skills.)

- **Work Skills:** My work skills at this time are:

(Example: Always on time, dress appropriately, get along with others, follow directions, have good physical strength, accept leadership)

_____	_____
_____	_____
_____	_____
_____	_____
_____	_____

- **Leisure Skills:** I enjoy doing the following:

(Ex: Physical sports such as basketball, social events, playing card games, travel)

_____	_____
_____	_____
_____	_____
_____	_____

(Put a check mark by those that you prefer more than others.)

- **Special Classes/Workshops attended and completed:**

(Example: Using computers, photography, art, dancing)

_____	_____
_____	_____
_____	_____
_____	_____
_____	_____

■ *Personal Assessment Information*

Throughout your schooling experience, as well as when you apply for employment or when you apply to advance in a career, taking some kind of test or inventory is usually required. It is recommended that you keep the information in order to help you in planning and advancing in a career of your choice, to get along with others, and to make key decisions. Remember: *This document is yours! Put in only the information you want.*

The following categories of assessment instruments allow for your interpretation.

- **LEARNING STYLE:**
- **Name of Survey:**_____

Results _____

_____

Interpretation _____

_____

■ Name of Survey:_____

Results _____

_____

Interpretation _____

_____

■ **ACHIEVEMENT:** _____

Results _____

_____

Interpretation _____

_____

_____

_____

■ **INTERESTS:** _____

Results _____

_____

Interpretation _____

_____

_____

_____

■ **VALUES:** _____

Results _____

_____

Interpretation _____

_____

_____

■ **SELF-ESTEEM:** _____

Results _____

_____

Interpretation _____

_____

_____

■ **OTHER:** _____

Results _____

_____

Interpretation _____

_____

■ *Current Resume*

Your resume is a description of you that describes your career (job) goals, your skills and training, and your recent work history for potential employers. It is a way to sell yourself, and usually accompanies your job application and a cover letter you have prepared to solicit employment. A resume usually contains information about you under four major headings: (1) Job Objective, (2) Skills and Abilities, (3) Experience, and (4) Education. It is important that you include *ALL* information relevant to the job for which you are applying. Prepare your resume and place it in the provided plastic holder. Remember: *You are to update your resume every year.*

Examples of Skills, Attitudes, and Abilities

accepts criticism well
accurate
adaptable
arbitrates
artistic
assembles
assertive
athletic ability
bilingual
builds things
careful
caring
catalogs
classifies
communication
computer skills
considerate
cooperative
creative
decision maker
dedicated
dependable
detail work
edits
energetic

enthusiastic
expedites
files
fixs things
flexible
follows directions
helping
honest
insightful
leadership
learn quickly
listening
logical
mathematical
motivated
neat
negotiates
operate machines
organizes
patient
people-oriented
performing arts
persuasive
precise
planning

problem solving
productive
punctual
reliable
resourceful
responds quickly
responsible
self-confident
self-motivated
selling
sets goals
takes initiative
teamwork
telephone skills
thorough
thoughtful
versatile
willing to change
multitasking
works with people
works steadily on one task
works well with hand tools
works well with others
works well by myself
writes well

Worksheet

Name _____

Address _____

Phone Number _____

Job Objective:

Work History:

Education:

Skills/Abilities:

References:

■ *Current Career Choice*

The Guidance Information System (GIS) is a computerized program that assists you in choosing a career and in developing plans to acquire the skills required. It is located in the Career Resource Center, the counselor's office, or the library. If you cannot locate it, please ask a counselor, administrator, or one of the secretaries. When you have found the system, do the following:

1. Make an appointment to use the program.
2. If you require assistance, please ask.
3. On completion, see your counselor immediately, and have the results explained; see if you are taking the appropriate classes in school; and decide on some learning experiences that will help you learn more of what is expected.
4. Place the results in the plastic envelope provided in this section.
5. Describe to your parents the results and how you plan to achieve your goals.

Remember: *You are expected to complete a career search in Grades 7, 9 and 11, at a minimum and are encouraged to use the college and career selection program each year.*

Career Information Inventories

— Setting Career Plans—

Date Taken	Careers	Date Discussed	Counselor Comments

Notes:

Date Taken	Careers	Date Discussed	Counselor Comments

Notes:

Date Taken	Careers	Date Discussed	Counselor Comments

Notes:

■ *College/University Application*

It is very important that you provide all information requested on college and university application forms. The information must also be correct and should be typed, unless otherwise directed. A form has been provided for your use and to provide some knowledge on what to expect.

Also provided is a holder for a copy of your personal essay required by some universities and colleges.

Remember: *Always keep copies of every application as well as letters, and essays sent!*

Your Record

Requests for Applications:

Name of School   Address   Date Sent   Date Received

_____

_____

_____

_____

_____

Applications Returned:

Acknowledgement   Name of School   Address   Date Sent   Date Received

_____

_____

_____

_____

Essay:
Completed on _____
Checked by _____
Retyped on _____
Checked by _____
Mailed on _____

Colleges Visited:
Name _____ Date _____
Name _____ Date _____
Name _____ Date _____
Name _____ Date _____
Name _____ Date _____

■ *Financial Aid Search*

A major activity required for all students to accomplish before the end of grade 11 is completion of a financial aid search. There is a computerized financial aid search program available at the high school. It will provide you with a list of options for consideration when you graduate from high school and plan to go on to a trade or technical school, a college, or a university.

To complete a search, you request an information form from the Guidance Office. The information requested requires some knowledge of your family and parents' background which you may not have. In this case, please see your counselor, contact your parents, or write them and send the form with instructions to fill it out and return it as soon as possible.

You are expected to complete the financial aid search at least twice during high school.

After the Search

After you have completed the financial aid search, please do the following:

1. Review all possibilities.
2. Select those for which you think you qualify.

3. Meet with and discuss the options with your counselor.

4. Send for all necessary information.

5. Alert your parents on what you are doing and that they may have to complete some forms as well as provide specific information.

6. Complete information, have it checked, mail.

Date Search(s) completed	Results	Discussed with Counselor	Date
_____	_____	_____	_____
_____	_____	_____	_____
_____	_____	_____	_____
_____	_____	_____	_____

Notes:

Put Copy of Search Results in Plastic Envelope for Future Use

■ *Letters of Recommendation and Commendation*

It is very important that you accumulate letters of recommendation and commendation as you prepare to make the transition from high school to more education, the armed services, work, or a combination of learning and working. The letters can be from teachers, employers, ministers, counselors, scout masters, and others who can validate your strengths. It may be difficult for you to request a letter, but this practice is very acceptable since most people are unaware that you would like one for your files.

The letter should provide some information about your skills, abilities, attitudes, and interpersonal relationships. Don't be afraid to say that you want the person to include information about your skills in ____, or your ability to ____, or your positive attitude toward others.

It is recommended that you have a minimum of one, and hopefully two letters, a year for grades 6–12. Yes, the more the better. Keep the originals, and when letters of reference are required, send a copy unless originals are requested. Keep an updated address on all people from whom you have letters so that if an updated letter is needed you know where to write or call.

References

List the name, address, and phone number of each person you want to use as a reference, including those from whom you already have a letter. Also, note when you knew the person and on what characteristics the person should write a recommendation or reference.

Name _____   Name _____

Address _____   Address _____

Phone _____   Phone _____

When did you know   When did you know
him/her _____   him/her _____

What characteristics   What characteristics
will they recommend _____   will they recommend _____

Name _____   Name _____

Address _____   Address _____

Phone _____   Phone _____

When did you know   When did you know
him/her _____   him/her _____

What characteristics   What characteristics
will they recommend _____   will they recommend _____

■ *Student Records*

The school is responsible for keeping track of the courses you take and the grades you achieve. School personnel also keep track of your attendance. *You* are responsible for making sure the school records are accurate. One way to do this is to keep track of your progress:

1. Write down the classes you take, the grades you receive, and the name of the teacher(s) of each class.

2. Keep copies of your report cards.

This document allows you to do both. There are forms for you to record your educational progress, and there is a plastic folder for you to keep copies of reports for future reference.

Your records are important, and it is your responsibility to maintain them and to make sure they are accurate.

If you have any questions, see your counselor immediately.

Record the courses you completed, the grades you achieved for each course, and the name of the teacher who taught each course completed.

School _____   Address _____

GRADE 9   FIRST SEMESTER
Course   Grade   Teacher

English _____

_____

_____

_____

_____

_____

Counselor _____

School _____   Address _____

GRADE 10   FIRST SEMESTER
Course   Grade   Teacher

English _____

_____

_____

_____

_____

_____

Counselor _____

School _____   Address _____

GRADE 11   FIRST SEMESTER
Course   Grade   Teacher

English _____

_____

_____

_____

_____

_____

Counselor _____

GRADE 9   SECOND SEMESTER
Course   Grade   Teacher

English _____

_____

_____

_____

_____

_____

Counselor _____

GRADE 10   SECOND SEMESTER
Course   Grade   Teacher

English _____

_____

_____

_____

_____

_____

Counselor _____

GRADE 11   SECOND SEMESTER
Course   Grade   Teacher

English _____

_____

_____

_____

_____

_____

Counselor _____

School _____   Address _____

GRADE 12   FIRST SEMESTER
Course   Grade   Teacher

English _____

_____

_____

_____

_____

_____

_____

Counselor _____

Graduated   Yes _____   No _____

GRADE 12   SECOND SEMESTER
Course   Grade   Teacher

English _____

_____

_____

_____

_____

_____

_____

Counselor _____

If yes, Date _____

Community Services

A major responsibility of all citizens is to contribute to the community in ways that are available, and possible. For example, you can volunteer to help in fundraising drives such as the Heart Fund, Red Cross, United Way, Homeless and Abused Children. You might volunteer to be a candy striper, to help with Meals on Wheels, or to give time and energy to the elderly living in nursing homes. scouting, peer tutoring, helping with team sports for the underprivileged, such as soccer, little league, or volleyball.

It is important and it is your responsibility to document your community service. Many colleges and universities now require evidence of community service contributions for admission. The evidence can include letters from appropriate people, notification of merit badges, pictures of you providing the services. There is a place on the back of this page for you to enter the community services you have provided and a plastic envelope for you to store your letters, and other documents.

Remember: *It is your responsibility to maintain a current and ongoing record of community service provided.*

Extra Curricular Activities

This is a place for you to record your extracurricular activities for future reference. This information not only shows what is important to you, but also may be required in future applications for schools, colleges, universities, and employment.

Please include as much information as possible. It may be necessary for you to ask your family members for specifics on what happened in grade school, places traveled, theater performances, art and other museums visited.

Remember: *You may want to ask the school counselor to review your school records to see if you have forgotten anything.*

EXTRACURRICULAR ACTIVITIES

Club Membership		Team Membership		Student Body Government	
Name	Dates	Name	Dates	Office	Dates

Travels		Performances		Museums/Art	
Country/State	When	Name	Date	Name	Date

Other:					
Name	Date	Name	Date	Name	Date

The following checklists are for your use to ensure that you know and take appropriate steps toward becoming a successful learner, worker, friend, and adult. When you have completed a competency, ask a responsible adult at school, at home, or in the community to initial and date the checklist to validate that you have successfully demonstrated the competency. Remember, this is for you to monitor your own progress.

Middle School

PURPOSE: The following checklist is used as a way to make sure that you have the competencies to develop educational and career goals and related decisions and plans. When you demonstrate specific competencies, your counselor, teacher, administrator, career resource technician, or parent can initial the record.

DATE	INITIALS	GRADE 6

CAREER/OCCUPATIONAL

_____ _____ I have identified my work interests.
_____ _____ I have examined work styles and my work interests.
_____ _____ I can list the elements of decision making.
_____ _____ I can identify potential jobs that I can do.
_____ _____ I can use the Career Resource Center materials correctly.

EDUCATIONAL

_____ _____ I know the school facilities and the resources.
_____ _____ I have knowledge of study skills.
_____ _____ I know students' rights and responsibilities.
_____ _____ I have knowledge of how to take tests.
_____ _____ I can list the elements of planning.

PERSONAL/SOCIAL

_____ _____ I can resolve interpersonal conflicts.
_____ _____ I know how to solve personal problems.
_____ _____ I know where to get help with personal problems.
_____ _____ _____
_____ _____ _____

DATE	INITIALS	GRADE 7

CAREER / OCCUPATIONAL

_____ _____ I can describe careers that match my work skills.
_____ _____ I can identify and use sources of career information.
_____ _____ I can demonstrate competencies needed to keep a job.
_____ _____ I can list the competencies needed to apply for a job.
_____ _____ I can identify the major elements of a career plan.
_____ _____ I can identify local work opportunities.

EDUCATIONAL

_____ _____ I can describe good study skills.
_____ _____ I can identify my academic strengths.
_____ _____ I am involved in at least one school-related extracurricular activity.
_____ _____ I can complete a written educational plan.
_____ _____ I can describe my learning style.

PERSONAL/SOCIAL

_____ _____ I have skills in resolving conflicts.
_____ _____ I have skills in making friends.
_____ _____ I can handle my own stress.
_____ _____ _____
_____ _____ _____

DATE	INITIALS	

GRADE 8
CAREER/OCCUPATIONAL

_____ _____ I can describe my work skills and match them with local job opportunities.
_____ _____ I have a tentative career plan matching my identified work skills and interests.
_____ _____ I can list occupations related to each of my current courses.
_____ _____ I have participated in career exploration activities.
_____ _____ I can list course offerings and career training opportunities in vocational education.
_____ _____ I can use the career decision-making process in choosing a career.

EDUCATIONAL

_____ _____ I can demonstrate good study skills.
_____ _____ I can demonstrate test-taking techniques.
_____ _____ I use my rights as a student as explained in the student handbook.
_____ _____ I show responsibility to others.
_____ _____ I have completed an educational plan for the ninth grade.
_____ _____ I have identified my aptitudes.
_____ _____ I can identify college/university entrance requirements.
_____ _____ I know the high school graduation requirements.

PERSONAL/SOCIAL

_____ _____ I know how my personality type effects others.
_____ _____ I know when and where to refer someone for help with personal problems.
_____ _____ _____
_____ _____ _____

Senior High School

PURPOSE: The following checklist is used as a way to make sure that you have the competencies to develop educational and career goals and related decisions and plans. When you demonstrate specific competencies, your counselor, teacher, administrator, career resource technician, or parent will initial the folder.

DATE	INITIALS	

GRADE 9
CAREER/OCCUPATIONAL

_____ _____ I can identify my tentative career goal. It is: _____
_____ _____ I can identify attitudes and skills for which employers look in job applicants.
_____ _____ I know how to use all the career information resources in the Career Resource Center.
_____ _____ I can use the career decision-making process in choosing a career.
_____ _____ I know my work traits and interests.

EDUCATIONAL

_____ _____ I have completed my Four-Year Educational Plan.
_____ _____ I know my academic strengths and learning style.
_____ _____ I can describe the educational program opportunities available to me.
_____ _____ I know my rights and responsibilities as a student and a citizen.
_____ _____ I can identify college/university entrance requirements.
_____ _____ I can identify technical/trade school entrance requirements.
_____ _____ I know the high school graduation requirements.

OTHER

_____ _____ _____
_____ _____ _____

DATE	INITIALS	GRADE 10

CAREER/OCCUPATIONAL

_____ _____ I can identify my tentative career goal. It is: _____

_____ _____ I can describe my work skills.

_____ _____ I can identify local job opportunities.

_____ _____ I can demonstrate job-seeking and application skills.

_____ _____ I can use at least four sources to find career/occupational information.

EDUCATIONAL

_____ _____ I have reviewed (and changed) my Four-Year Educational Plan.

_____ _____ I can describe my academic competencies.

_____ _____ I know how to plan for long-range goals.

OTHER

_____ _____ _____

_____ _____ _____

DATE	INITIALS	GRADE 11

CAREER/OCCUPATIONAL

_____ _____ I can identify my tentative career goal. It is: _____

_____ _____ I am in a course of study that leads to my career goal.

_____ _____ I can demonstrate positive job-interviewing skills.

EDUCATIONAL

_____ _____ I have reviewed my high school plan.

_____ _____ I have discussed my current educational plans with my counselor and my parents.

OTHER

_____ _____ _____

_____ _____ _____

DATE	INITIALS	GRADE 12

CAREER/OCCUPATIONAL

_____ _____ I can identify my tentative career goal. It is: _____

_____ _____ I have had one or more work/leisure/educational experiences outside of school that relate to my career goal.

_____ _____ I have a written plan for reaching my career goal.

EDUCATIONAL

_____ _____ After high school, I plan to ____.

_____ _____ I have taken the following action on my post–high school plan____.

_____ _____ I have discussed my post–high school plans with my counselor and parents.

OTHER

_____ _____ _____

_____ _____ _____

_____ _____ _____

■ *Senior High School: Grades 9–12 Competencies*

PURPOSE: The following checklist is used as a way to make sure that you have the competencies to develop educational and career goals and to make related decisions and plans. When you demonstrate specific competencies, your counselor, teacher, administrator, Career Technician, or parent will initial the folder.

DATE	INITIALS	GRADE 9

CAREER/OCCUPATIONAL

_____ _____ I can identify my tentative career goal. It is _____
_____ _____ I can identify attitudes and skills employers want from employees.
_____ _____ I know how to use all the career information resources in the Career Center.
_____ _____ I can use the career decision-making process in choosing a career.

EDUCATIONAL COMPETENCIES

_____ _____ I have completed my Four-Year Educational Plan.
_____ _____ I know my academic strengths and learning style.
_____ _____ I can describe the educational program opportunities available to me.
_____ _____ I know my rights and responsibilities as a student and a citizen.
_____ _____ I can identify college/university entrance requirements.
_____ _____ I can identify technical/trade school entrance requirements.
_____ _____ I know the high school graduation requirements.

DATE	INITIALS	GRADE 10

CAREER/OCCUPATIONAL

I can identify my tentative career goal. It is: _____
_____ _____ I can describe my work skills.
_____ _____ I can identify local job opportunities.
_____ _____ I can demonstrate job-seeking and application skills
_____ _____ I can use at least four sources to find careeer/occupational information.

EDUCATIONAL COMPETENCIES

I have reviewed (and changed) my Four-Year Educational Plan.
_____ _____ I can describe my academic competencies.
_____ _____ I know how to plan for long-range goals.
_____ _____

DATE	INITIALS	GRADE 11

CAREER/OCCUPATIONAL

_____ _____ I can identify my tentative career goal. It is _____
_____ _____ I am in a course of study that leads to my career goal.
_____ _____ I can demonstrate positive job-interviewing skills.

EDUCATIONAL COMPETENCIES

_____ _____ I have reviewed (and revised) my high school plan.
_____ _____ I have discussed my educational plans with my counselor and my parents.

DATE	INITIALS	
		GRADE 12
		CAREER/OCCUPATIONAL
_____	_____	I can identify my tentative career goal. It is _____
_____	_____	I have had one or more work/leisure/educational experiences outside of school that relate to my career goal
_____	_____	I have a written plan for reaching my career goal.
		EDUCATIONAL COMPETENCIES
_____	_____	After high school, I plan to _____
_____	_____	I have taken the following action on my post high school plan _____
_____	_____	I have discussed my post high school plans with my counselor and parents.

■ *Counselor's Logs*

Please use the counselor's log to record your sessions with the counselor. Make notes on instructions or suggestions that the counselor provides. By tracking the dates, you can be assured that you have maintained contact and are meeting all timelines toward graduation and meeting post–high school goals.

COUNSELOR'S LOG
Parent Contacts

DATE	CONTENT	RESPONSE	PHONE MAIL

COUNSELOR'S LOG

Student Conference

DATE	COMMENTS	PLAN	FOLLOW-UP DATE

Sample Performance Evaluation Form

The shift from counseling services to student support programs calls for a different means to evaluate professional performance. In the traditional approach, the performance evaluation of counselors and other student support personnel often used the teacher evaluation form listing a set of tasks (role and function) on which the evaluation was based. In the results-based program, a shift has been made to use the performance evaluation as a dual responsibility of the administrator and the counselor. Evaluation is defined as a process of using information to improve the quantity and quality of the program. Therefore, the counselor or other student support professional evaluates his or her program contributions, reflects on each result, and projects what he/she plans to do differently. This self report is then forwarded to the administrator in charge who will review the document, call a meeting to discuss the contributions and reflections of the professional, and express appreciation of the efforts. It is during this time that the administrator can add suggestions for modification of proposed changes as well as identify planned activities that may need to be modified or even dropped and replaced by something else that more closely matches the school's goals and directions for the following year. This is a consensus building process—the professional counselor evaluates himself or herself and shares the results, reflections, and plans with the administrator who in turn appreciates and find ways to help facilitate the future plans.

A Developmental Continuum of Counselor Contributions: Counselor Assessment and Support Program

September 2000

Skills Needed for The Comprehensive, Results-Based Guidance Program
Aligned with the California Counselor Leadership Academy and
ASCA National Standards for School Counseling Programs

Developed by C.D. Johnson, Ph.D., and Sharon Johnson, Ed.D.

■ *Rubrics Counselor Competencies*

OVERVIEW: **Results-Based Guidance Program** Plans, organizes, delivers, and evaluates a comprehensive results-based guidance program that impacts all students in academic achievement, career planning, and personal social development.

Minimal Criteria for Success:

■ Submits results agreement that includes student results, personal development results, parent results, staff development results, and other assigned tasks.

■ Results agreement is negotiated and approved by the administrator.

■ Develops and submits program plan that includes student competencies to be attained, content, activities, timeline, person responsible, materials, and evaluation strategies.

1.0 Results Agreement: Submits results agreement that includes student results, personal development results, parent results, staff development results and other assigned tasks.

Not Operational	Needs Improvement	Operational	Excellent	Exemplary
• Results agreement is incomplete or unacceptable to administrator. • Little evidence of collaboration with team members or others involved in delivery of results. • Results agreement is missing elements such as results for parents, staff, and personal growth. • Plans are sketchy, unclear, or incomplete. • Planned activities do not address all students.	• Results agreement includes most of the defined elements but may be unclear. • Plans include activities to address all students but do not include others in delivery of results. • Administrator needs assistance to clearly understand results agreement and plans and only conditionally approves.	• Results agreement includes all defined elements at an understandable level but may need some interpretation for clarity and exactness. • Plans are complete and include minimal collaboration with others involved in delivery of results. • Results agreement and plans are submitted on time, are comprehensive, and address all students based on specified student results but may lack detailed planning.	• Results agreement include all defined elements, are clear and understandable to counselors, teachers, and administrators. • Results agreement and plans are submitted on time. • There is evidence of collaboration with others in the development of plans. • Results and plans demonstrate detailed planning of activities to address all students in delivery of results.	• Results agreement includes all defined elements, are submitted on time, are neat and complete. • Results agreement is clearly defined and easily understood by administrators, teachers, parents, and community members. • Results agreement and plans are based on school/district data. • Program plans are developed in collaboration with all others involved in delivery of results and proactively address all students.

Program Plans: Results Agreement

Counselor's Contributions

Evidence	Reflections

Administrator's Observations

Evidence	Reflections

Results Agreement

1.1 Program Results:

Not Operational	Needs Improvement	Operational	Excellent	Exemplary
Written in terms of what the counselor will do or what activities will be done for an unspecified population.	Written in terms of process or activity results for a specific population in a specific domain or for a specific goal.	Defines student results in evaluable competencies for a specific population related to a guidance goal.	Defines student results in evaluable competencies for a specific population and is directly related to student achievement and to specific guidance goals.	Defines student results in evaluable competencies for all students (or a specific caseload), in a specific domain or goal as it relates to school and district goals, student achievement, and school/district data.

Counselor Comments

Evidence	Reflections

Administrator Observations

Evidence	Reflections

1.2 Parent Results:

Not Operational	Needs Improvement	Operational	Excellent	Exemplary
Parent-based results are not included in the results agreement.	Parent results are stated in terms of activities, number of contacts, or processes.	Parent results are stated in terms of specific competencies parents will acquire.	Parent results are stated in terms of specific competencies parents will acquire related to student academic achievement. Results are planned for all parents.	Parent results are stated for a specific population, include specific competencies related to students' academic, career, and college plans, and personal/social adjustment; are planned for all parents.

Counselor Comments

Evidence	Reflections

Administrator Observations

Evidence	Reflections

1.3 Staff Results:

Not Operational	Needs Improvement	Operational	Excellent	Exemplary
Staff results are not included in the results agreement.	Staff results are stated in terms of what teachers will receive through participation in a counselor directed activity or inservice.	Staff results are stated in terms of competencies staff will acquire that relate to the guidance goals/ results for students.	Staff results are stated for a specific group of staff members who will acquire competencies to facilitate student achievement.	Staff results are stated in terms of specific, identified competencies for identified staff members to ensure student academic achievement and successful student plans for college/ career.

Counselor Comments

Evidence	Reflections

Administrator Observations

Evidence	Reflections

1.4 Self-Improvement:

Not Operational	Needs Improvement	Operational	Excellent	Exemplary
Self-improvement results are not included in the results agreement.	Self-improvement results are written in terms of what the counselor hopes to do (not necessarily what they will learn or skills they will acquire).	Identifies specific counseling and guidance-related competencies to be acquired.	Identifies specific counselor competencies to be acquired that relate directly to implementing the guidance program goals.	Identifies specific counselor competencies to be acquired that are directly related to facilitating the student-based results, academic achievement, and/or staff or parent development.

Counselor Comments

Evidence	Reflections

Administrator Observations

Evidence	Reflections

Program Plan: Implementation

2.0 Implementation Plan: Develops and submits program plan that includes student competencies to be attained, content, activities, timeline, person responsible, materials, and evaluation strategies.

Not Operational	Needs Improvement	Operational	Excellent	Exemplary
• Little preparation is evident in plan for implementation. • Plan appears disorganized or incomplete. • Does not include team members or other persons who can add to the quality of the plan.	• Indicates limited materials within plan. • Limited effort in planning time for activities or in use of appropriate and varied instructional approaches. • Evaluates number of students, parents, or staff who participate.	• Develops/acquires materials to deliver student results. • Completes schedule of events for implementation including competencies to be delivered, specific content to be included, who is responsible for each task, activities and materials to be used, where and when activities will occur, means of evaluation, and criteria of success.	• Develops comprehensive plan for delivery of specific student competencies. • Arranges to pilot test and make necessary changes in timing, instruction, and/or materials and equipment based on results of initial trial. • Collects data on pilot test and uses them in making revisions.	• Uses developed materials with appropriate instructional activities to impact the planned specific student population. • Shows competent time management skills. • Schedules follow-through contact with students requiring additional assistance. • Coordinates plan with other staff members. • Provides feedback to team members and teaching staff as appropriate. • Meets with administration to share results and reflections.

Implementation Plan

Counselor Comments

Evidence	Reflections

Administrator Observations

Evidence	Reflections

Program Evaluation

3.0 Evaluating Program Effectiveness:

Not Operational	Needs Improvement	Operational	Excellent	Exemplary
• Does not document evidence of student acquiring specific competencies.	• Evaluates in terms of the number of students (staff and/or parents) who participated in an activity or who received information.	• Evaluates student attainment of results using preestablished criteria and methods to collect data. • Shares results with guidance team.	• Uses the data to show contributions to guidance and school goal achievement and to impact on other school profile elements such as failures, truants, referrals, etc. • Shares data with staff.	• Uses data in planning and implementing strategies for improvement of program activities. • Has a written reflection on the successes and means to increase results.

Counselor Comments

Evidence	Reflections

Administrator Observations

Evidence	Reflections

4.0 Monitoring: Monitors all students' academic progress and intervenes with students who are not meeting educational expectations.

Minimal Criteria for Success:

- Monitors each assigned student's academic progress a minimum of every six weeks.

- Identifies students requiring assistance and determines what is needed by each, e.g., study skills, homework preparation, parent-teacher conference, study rituals at home, notetaking skills, tutoring, etc.

- Develops and implements plans for each student not meeting academic expectations.

- Maintains monitoring until student achievement is meeting expectancy.

Not Operational	Needs Improvement	Operational	Excellent	Exemplary
Uses report cards and teacher referral to monitor progress and to identify students in need of help. • Mails home notice of deficiency or failure.	• Has an individual conference with each student in the assigned caseload to warn them of the results of failing or not working up to expectations. • Establishes means for monitoring student progress for purpose of reporting information to the administrator and parent.	• Monitors each assigned student's academic progress a minimum of every six weeks. • Holds a conference with student to determine a course of action for improvement. • Contacts parent/guardian to alert them to potential problems.	Meets all criteria listed under Operational Level plus: • Identifies students requiring assistance and determines what is needed by each to increase achievement, e.g., study skills, homework preparations, parent-teacher-student conference, etc. • Develops a plan with each student. • Establishes appointment times for feedback and monitoring. • Establishes communication with teachers and parents to track student progress.	• Identified students needing assistance who have a plan for improvement will have a conference with each teacher to establish what can be done. • Each student will develop career and educational plans and a career portfolio. • Each teacher is contacted and requested to supply ongoing information on specific student's progress. • Team meeting with student, parent, teachers is held to determine an effective system to monitor student's progress until achievement improves.

Monitoring Student Progress

Counselor Comments

Evidence	Reflections

Administrator Observations

Evidence	Reflections

5.0 Advocacy: Uses advocacy skills with teachers and parents to ensure understanding and agreement on appropriate developmental progress.

Minimal Criteria for Success:

- Establishes effective professional relationships and consults with staff on student and school issues and programs.
- Shares student information with staff, within the limits of confidentiality.
- Consults with parents/guardians and staff regarding students' academic, career and personal/social development.
- Serves as an effective liaison between the school, district and community agencies.
- Interprets the comprehensive results-based guidance program and expectations to students, staff, parents, and community.

Not Operational	Needs Improvement	Operational	Excellent	Exemplary
• No evidence of student advocacy outside of assigned duties.	• Meets with student individually to determine student needs, plans, grades, and personal/social issues.	• Consults with staff on student and school issues and programs. • Consults with parents/guardians and staff regarding students' academic, career, personal/social, and wellness development. • Interprets the comprehensive, results-based guidance program and expectations to students, staff, parents, and community.	• Meets all criteria listed under Operational Level. • Establishes effective professional relationships with staff, parents, and community members. • Mentors other adults in learning how to facilitate student achievement, including tutoring and community service. • Shares appropriate information with staff to facilitate student achievement.	• Meets all criteria listed under Operational and Excellent Levels. • Shows evidence of advocacy with each student in assigned caseload. • Has scheduled conferences with each student's parent/guardians regarding career and post–high school educational plans. • Conducts case conference for each student in need of support.

Advocacy

Counselor Comments

Evidence	Reflections

Administrator Observations

Evidence	Reflections

6.0 Counseling Skills: Uses applicable guidance and counseling techniques appropriately to facilitate academic, career, and personal/social results.

Minimal Criteria for Success:

- Uses a variety of guidance competencies, techniques, and strategies to enhance student learning, e.g., assessment, learning-teaching style match, extra-curricular involvement, parent involvement, student support team consultation, etc.

- Uses counseling skills to facilitate students personal problem solving.

- Interprets accurately standardized test results to students, parents, staff, and community.

- Plans educational progress in collaboration with students and their parents that are commensurate with their needs, goals, and abilities.

- Establishes and maintains good rapport with students, parents, and staff.

- Conducts group counseling and group guidance activities; provides classroom guidance activities; and uses individual, parent, and group conferencing skillfully to attain positive results.

Evidence	Reflections

7.0 Professional Renewal: Continues to renew and acquire professional competencies applicable to school counseling.

- Continues to renew and acquire new professional competencies.
- Is actively involved in counselor professional growth activities such as professional workshops, conferences, publishing, research, etc.
- Keeps updated on current practices, theories, issues, and trends in student support programs.
- Demonstrates sensitivity to needs of minorities and community members.
- Demonstrates self-motivation, team membership, and leadership.

Evidence	Reflections

8.0 Other Professional Contributions:

Staff Relationships:

- Collaborates with others to accomplish program goals.
- Participates in regularly scheduled staff meetings, department meetings, school staff events.
- Establishes rapport with staff members.
- Consults with psychologists, CWAs, teachers, administrators about individual students.

Staff Responsibilities:

- Assumes an active role as a staff member.
- Participates on school instructional and supplemental services teams (SST, Special Education screening, etc.).
- Utilizes established channels for positive change.
- Communicates guidance goals to administrators and staff members.
- Punctual in submitting paperwork, appointments and other time commitments.

Evidence	Reflections

■ *Summary Report of Results*

After carefully reviewing results, evidence collected, and reflections, the following summary and suggestions are identified for consideration and discussion:

	Counselor	Administrator
Strengths		
Weaknesses		
Suggested Changes		

Sample Management Flowchart for Developing a Results-Based Student Support Program

The flowchart is a visual representation of how a program may be developed.

1. The rectangle represents a product or a process.

2. The diamond represents a decision-making activity.

3. The small circles represent connectors: the circle with a **dot** in the middle is used to say that **all** activities following will be completed; the circle with a **+** in the middle is used when the person or team has a choice of doing **one or more** of the tasks; and the circle with / in the middle directs that **only one choice** can be made of the identified alternatives.

The flowchart identifies each element in sequence and indicates that when consensus is reached by the team or individual designing the element, the administrator is asked to review and approve, request more information, or ask for a revision. Once the administrator agrees, then the subsequent element is developed. This process of consensus seeking must be followed for each element of the program. The end product, a results-based student/guidance support program, is then ready for implementation.

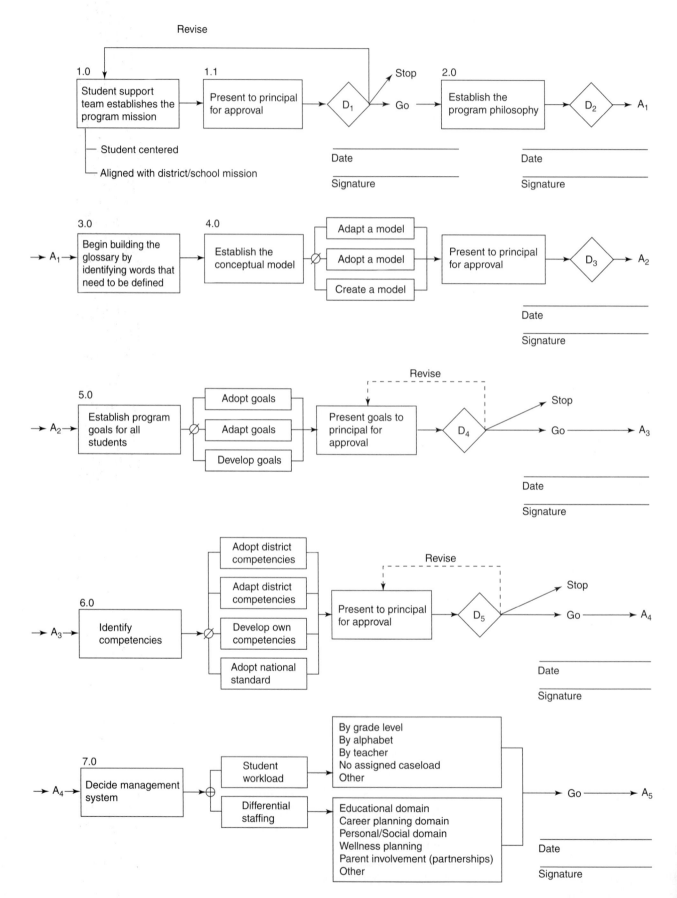

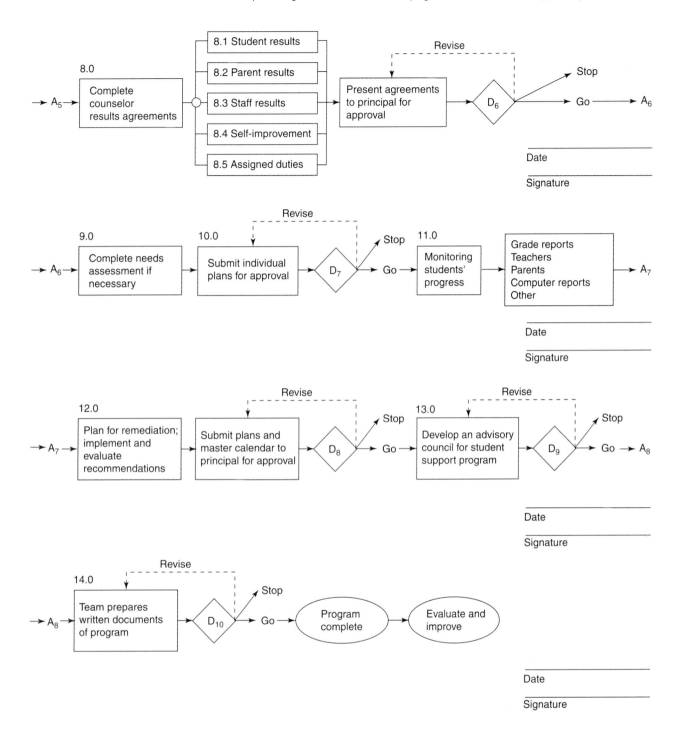

References

American School Counselor Association (2003). *The ASCA national model: A framework for school counseling programs.* Alexandria, VA: Author.

Anderson, R. (1989). *Mentoring.* Raleigh, NC: Wake County Public Schools.

Aubrey, R. (1989). *Counseling at the crossroad: Obstacles, opportunities, and options.* Ann Arbor: MI: ERIC/CAPS, School of Education, University of Michigan.

Barker, J. (1987). *Discovering the future: The business of paradigms.* (Videotape). Minneapolis, MN: Filmedia, Inc.

Beale, A. (2001). Emerging career development theories: A test for school counselors. *Professional School Counseling, 5,* 1–5.

Bemak, F. (2000). Transforming the role of the counselor to provide leadership in educational reform through collaboration. *Professional School Counseling, 3,* 323–331.

Bemak, F., & Cornely, L. (2002). The SAFI model as a critical link between marginalized families and schools: A literature review and strategies for school counselors. *Journal of Counseling and Development, 80,* 322–331.

Bradley, O. (1986). The effects of the Teacher-Advisor System on the students of Omaha Technical High School, Omaha, Nebraska, in the areas of attitude, attendance, behavior, and achievement. Unpublished doctoral dissertation. University of Nebraska, Lincoln. *Dissertation Abstracts International, 468–A,* 2139.

Campbell, C.A., & Dahir, C.A. (1997). *Sharing the vision: The national standards for school counseling programs.* Alexandria, VA: American School Counselor Association Press.

Drucker, P. (1971). What we can learn from Japanese management. *Executive Development Series, Part III.* Cambridge, MA: Harvard College.

Feller, R. (2003). Connecting school counseling to the current reality. *Professional School Counseling, 6,* ii-v.

Finn, C. (1990). The biggest reform of all. *Phi Delta Kappan, 71* (8), 584–592.

Gallassi, J., & Gulledge, S. (1997). The middle school counselor and teacher advisor programs. *Professional School Counseling, 1,* 55–60.

Gysbers, N. (2003). Comprehensive school guidance programs in the future: Staying the course. In C.D. Johnson & S. Johnson (Eds.), *Building stronger school counseling programs: Bringing futuristic approaches into the present* (pp. 145–153). Greensboro, NC: CAPS Publications.

Gysbers, N., & Henderson, P. (1988). *Developing and managing your school guidance program.* Alexandria, VA: American Association of Counseling and Development.

Hayslip, J. (2000). Using national standards and models of excellence as frameworks for accountability. *Journal of Career Development, 27,* 81–87.

Henderson, P. (1989). The role of the middle school counselor in teacher-advisor programs. *School Counselor, 36,* 348–351.

Herr, E. (1989). *Guidance and counseling: A shared responsibility.* Prepared for The Lilly Endowment, Indianapolis, Indiana.

Herr, E. (2002, April). School reform and perspectives on the role of school counselors: A century of proposals for change. *Professional School Counseling, 5,* 1–16.

House, R., & Hayes, R. (2002). Becoming key players in school reform. *Professional School Counseling, 5,* 249–256.

Hoyt, K. (1989). *Counselors and career development—a topic in education reform proposals: A selected review of national education reform documents.* Columbus, OH: Center on Education and Training for Employment, Ohio State University.

The Individuals with Disabilities Education Act of 1997, S. 105-17, 105th Cong., 1st Sess. (1997).

Ireh, M. (2000). Career development theories and their implications for high school career guidance and counseling. *High School Journal, 83,* 28–40.

Isaacs, M., (2003). Data-driven decision making: The engine of accountability. *Professional School Counseling, 6,* 288–295.

Jarvis, P., & Keeley, E. (2003). From vocational decision making to career building: Blueprint, real games, and school counseling. *Professional School Counseling, 6,* 244–251.

Johnson, C. (1988). *Career ladders: Breaking out of the mold of roles and functions.* Unpublished document. San Juan Capistrano, CA: Professional Update.

Johnson, C., & Johnson, S. (1982). Competency-based training of career development specialists or "lets get off the calf path." *Vocational Guidance Quarterly, 32,* 327–335.

Johnson, C., & Johnson, S. (1998). *California Counselor Leadership Academy Manual.* San Juan Capistrano, CA: Professional Update.

Johnson, S., & Ammon, T. (1994). The Arizona experience: A statewide approach to implementing competency-based guidance programs for all students. *Arizona Counselors Association Journal, 19,* 45–51.

Johnson, S., & Johnson, C.D. (1991). The new guidance: A systems approach to pupil personnel programs. *California Association of Counseling and Development Journal, 2,* 5–14.

Johnson, S., & Whitfield, E. (Eds.). (1991). *Evaluating guidance programs: A practitioner's guide.* Iowa: American College Testing Company.

Kaplan, L. (2000). Hiring the best school counseling candidates to promote achievement. *NASSP Bulletin, 83,* 34–39.

Kasler, M. (1989). A study to compare and contrast two types of student guidance delivery systems — with counselors and guidance resource technicians. Unpublished doctoral dissertation, Pepperdine University, 1988. *Dissertation Abstracts International,* 505–A, 1219.

Kaufman, R. (1972). *Educational system planning.* Englewood, NJ: Prentice-Hall.

Kiersey, D., & Bates, M. (1973). *Results system management.* Monograph No 3. Fullerton, CA: California Personnel and Guidance Association.

Kuhn, T. (1970). *The structure of scientific revolutions* (2nd ed.). Chicago: University of Chicago Press.

Lapan, R. (2001). Results-base comprehensive guidance and counseling programs: A framework for planning and evaluation. *Professional School Counseling, 4,* 289. (Document Reproduction Service No. CG031541)

Martin, P., & House, R. (1998). *Transforming school counseling in the transforming school counseling initiative.* Washington, DC: The Education Trust.

Mitchell, G., Udow, G., Downs, L., McMaster, S., DeWitt, K., Stevenson, M., Pares, C., & Sampson, L. (2002). *Do inland southern California schools meet American School Counselor Association national standards: A qualitative study.* (ERIC Document Reproduction Service No. ED467345)

Myrick, L., & Myrick, R. (1992). The teacher advisor program. In G. Walz & T. Ellis (Eds.), *Counseling and guidance in the schools: Three exemplary guidance approaches.* Washington, DC: National Education Association (pp. 25–44).

Myrick, R. (2003). *Developmental guidance and counseling: A practical approach* (4th ed.). Minneapolis, MN: Education Media Corp.

Myrick, R., & Myrick, L. (1990). *The teacher-advisor program: An innovative approach to school guidance.* Ann Arbor: MI: ERIC/CAPS, School of Education.

Nailor, P., & Squier, K. (2004). Data-driven without driving yourself crazy. *The School Counselor, 41* (3), 24–29.

Rowley, W., Sink, C., & MacDonald, G. (2002). An experiential and systemic approach to encourage collaboration and community building. *Professional School Counseling, 5,* 360–365.

Schwallie-Giddis, P., & Mercedes, P. (2003). Initiating leadership by introducing and implementing the ASCA national model. *Professional School Counseling, 6,* 170–173.

Senge, P. (1990). *The fifth discipline: The art & practice of the learning organization.* New York: Currency Doubleday.

Senge, P. (2000). *Schools that learn: A fifth discipline fieldbook for educators, parents and everyone who cares about education.* New York: Currency Doubleday.

Steinberg, L. (1988). Preparation of school counselors for the 1990's. *California Association for Counseling and Development Journal. 9*, 7–17.

Stone, C., & Dyal, M. (1997). School counselors sowing the seeds of character education. *Professional School Counseling, 1*, 22–24.

Walz, G. (1992). Putting it all together: Three exemplary guidance approaches. In G. Walz & T. Ellis (Eds.), *Counseling and guidance in the schools:* Washington, DC: National Education Association (pp. 61–69).

Wellman, F. (1964). *The national study of guidance taxonomy of objectives*. Monograph No. 3.

Fullerton, CA: California Personnel and Guidance Association.

White, R. (1981). *Guaranteed services for counseling and guidance: A model for program development*. San Jose, CA: Santa Clara County Office of Education.

TECHNOLOGY RESOURCE

Sabella, R. (2003). *School counselor.com 2.0: A friendly and practical guide to the world wide web*. Minneapolis, MN: Educational Media Corporation. (1,200+ counseling related websites)